Understanding Anxiety and Panic Attacks

Bradley Steffens

ReferencePoint Press

San Diego, CA

ReferencePoint Press®

For more information, contact:
ReferencePoint Press, Inc.
PO Box 27779
San Diego, CA 92198
www.ReferencePointPress.com

LIBRARY OF CONGRESS CATALOGING-IN-PUBLICATION DATA

Name: Steffens, Bradley- author
Title: Understanding Anxiety and Panic Attacks/by Bradley Steffens
Description: San Diego, CA: ReferencePoint Press, Inc, 2027. | Includes bibliographical references and index.
Identifiers: LCCN 2026010831 (print) | ISBN 978-1-6782-1376-3 library binding | ISBN 978-1-6782-1377-0 ebook
Subjects: LCSH: Juvenile literature

For compete cataloging-in-publication data please go to www.loc.gov.

CONTENTS

An Overwhelming Feeling

Many students feel anxiety when taking their final exams, knowing that their semester's grade may be on the line. This was the case for twenty-three-year-old Judith A. Verduzco, a student at California State University, Northridge. She was nervous before the exam, but without warning, her pretest jitters morphed into something terrifying:

> I was sitting in a Chicano Studies class, taking a final exam, when suddenly I felt an overwhelming wave of fear. My heart pounded, my chest tightened, and the room began to spin. . . . I vividly remember looking up at my professor and asking if I could step outside. He must have seen the terrified look on my face because he sent his aide to walk with me. I told her, "I don't feel well—I think I'm going to die." They called an ambulance, and in that moment, I was convinced I was having a heart attack.

> **"I was sitting in a Chicano Studies class, taking a final exam, when suddenly I felt an overwhelming wave of fear. My heart pounded, my chest tightened, and the room began to spin."[1]**
>
> —Judith A. Verduzco, a student at California State University, Northridge

Once at the hospital, Verduzco underwent a battery of medical tests. Hours later the test results came back. Everything was normal physically. "I was told I was fine," Verduzco recalls. The doctor explained that her physical symptoms—the pounding heart and shortness of breath—were all caused by her brain. "That was the first time I heard the words: panic attack,"[1] she says.

Serious Symptoms

The phrase *panic attack* is sometimes used in conversation—often lightheartedly—to describe momentary confusion or urgent concern. "I was having a panic attack,"[2] singer/songwriter Clinton Kane joked to his record producer, describing his sudden need to talk about one of his recordings. But a real panic attack is far from a laughing matter.

The physical symptoms of a panic attack can include rapid heart rate, sweating, trembling, shortness of breath, tightness in the throat, chills, numbness or tingling sensations, hot flashes, nausea, abdominal cramping, chest pain, headache, dizziness, lightheadedness, or faintness. These symptoms are completely real. In fact, the Mayo Clinic advises that a person experiencing such symptoms should seek immediate medical help because

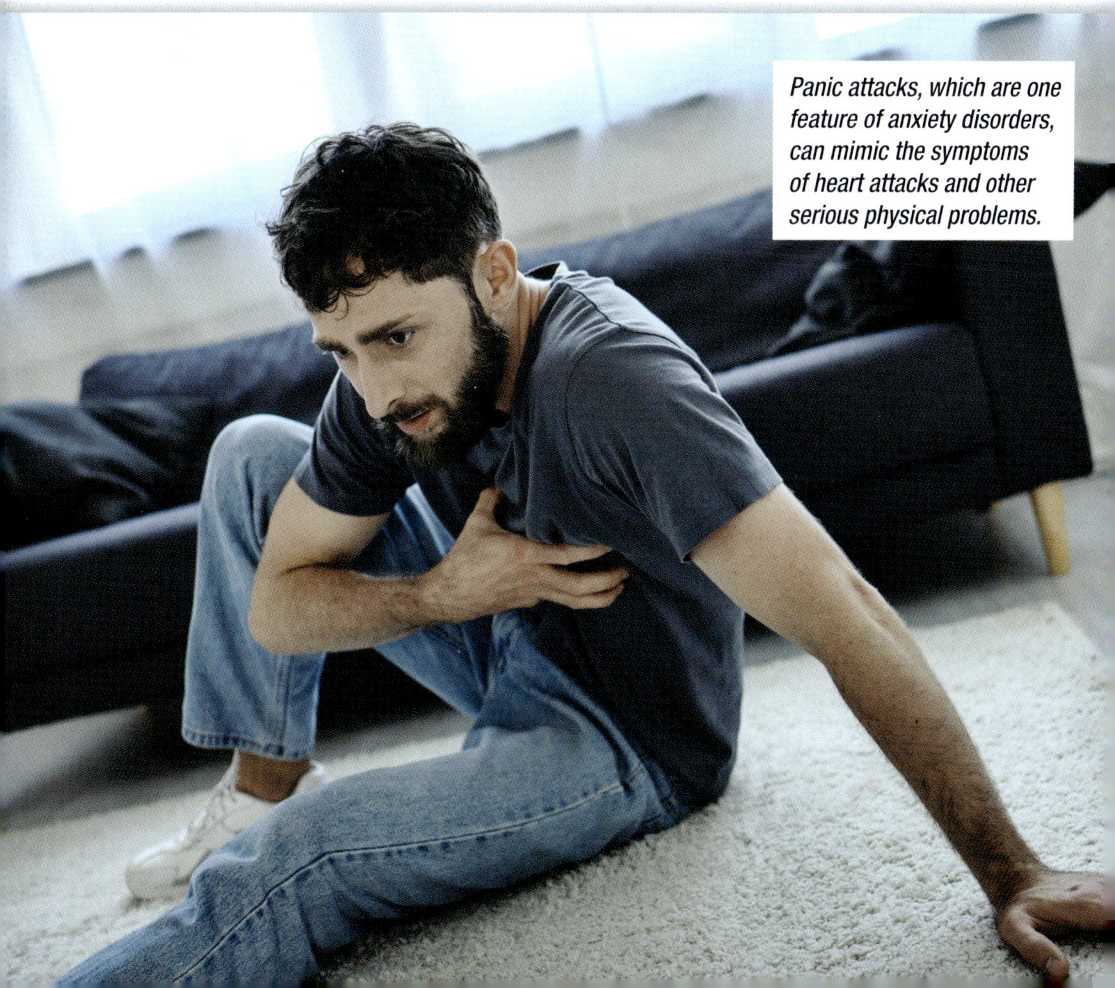

Panic attacks, which are one feature of anxiety disorders, can mimic the symptoms of heart attacks and other serious physical problems.

"Panic attack symptoms can also resemble symptoms of other serious health problems, such as a heart attack, so it's important to get evaluated."[3]

—Mayo Clinic

"panic attack symptoms can also resemble symptoms of other serious health problems, such as a heart attack, so it's important to get evaluated."[3]

Once a person has had a panic attack, they can often face a new problem: the intense fear that they will have another one. They may start to avoid situations they think could trigger another panic attack. When people alter their daily activities to avoid future panic attacks, they are suffering from what is known as panic disorder.

Anxiety Disorders

Panic disorder is one of several disorders in the broad category of what is known as anxiety disorders. According to the *Diagnostic and Statistical Manual of Mental Disorders, 5th Edition, Text Revision (DSM-5-TR)*, the handbook used by mental health professionals in the United States and worldwide to classify and diagnose mental disorders, to be diagnosed with an anxiety disorder, a person's worry or fear must meet two basic criteria: It must be out of proportion to the situation, and it must hinder the person's ability to function normally. In addition, the condition must persist over time, which the *DSM-5-TR* defines as occurring more days than not for at least six months. Everyone is different, so it is not surprising that there are different kinds of anxiety disorders. Some of the most common types are generalized anxiety disorder (GAD), panic disorder, social anxiety disorder, separation anxiety disorder, and phobias.

A Common Problem

According to the World Health Organization, more than a quarter of the global population experiences anxiety disorders at some point in their lives. The National Institute of Mental Health (NIMH) reports that anxiety disorders are the most widespread mental health challenge in the United States, affecting more than 42 million adults each year. Millions of teens are affected as well. NIMH studies have found that 31.9 percent of American adolescents have had an anxiety disorder by the time they reach age eighteen.

The good news is that anxiety disorders are highly treatable. A treatment known as cognitive behavioral therapy (CBT) often works wonders with anxiety patients. Other sufferers may respond to medications prescribed by a doctor. Adopting a balanced diet, getting moderate exercise, and having good sleep habits can also significantly affect anxiety disorders. Such lifestyle changes can reduce symptoms, boost well-being, and even prevent anxiety by influencing brain function, stress regulation, and overall emotional resilience. Millions of people suffer from anxiety, but they are able to manage it and lead fulfilling lives.

CHAPTER ONE

What Is Anxiety?

Anxiety is a feeling of unease, worry, or fear about future events. Everyone feels anxious at times—before a test, during a job interview, or before giving a presentation or speech, for example. The heart races. The stomach feels queasy. Breathing becomes rapid. These feelings are normal. They are the body's way of preparing a person to confront challenges. In small doses, anxiety is simply a signal that a person is facing something significant to them. "Instead of treating anxiety like an enemy to defeat, I began to see it as a message," writes blogger Glory Emmanuel. "Because the more I thought about it, the more I realized: Anxiety is just a signal that something matters to me."[4]

> "The more I thought about it, the more I realized: Anxiety is just a signal that something matters to me."[4]
>
> —Glory Emmanuel, mental health blogger

Fear of the Unknown

People feel anxiety about the future because it is unknown. No one feels anxious about the past. People may feel regret about the past, but they do not feel anxious about it, because it is over with and therefore known. And the more important a future event is to a person, the greater their anxiety will be. "We worry about . . . things we care about," observes sports psychologist Jonah Oliver. "I didn't get nervous making breakfast this morning."[5]

Even people who are used to facing pressure situations, such as professional athletes, still feel anxiety. "Oh, for sure I have anxiety," says ten-time National Basketball Association all-star and four-time champion Stephen Curry. "A lot of it is baked into the expectations I've set and the level I want to play at. . . . It's a healthy insecurity of having to prove yourself every single night, which is cool. It keeps you going."[6]

Improving Performance

A moderate amount of anxiety actually boosts performance by increasing focus, motivation, and alertness. This is known as optimal anxiety. Optimal anxiety prepares the body and mind for action, signaling the brain that the task at hand is important and sharpening attention to it. Anxiety can also trigger the release of a natural chemical in the brain called dopamine. The release of dopamine motivates a person to act and prepare to avoid negative outcomes. The mixture of effort and anxiety can create what is known as a flow state, a mental outlook that leads to peak experiences and performance.

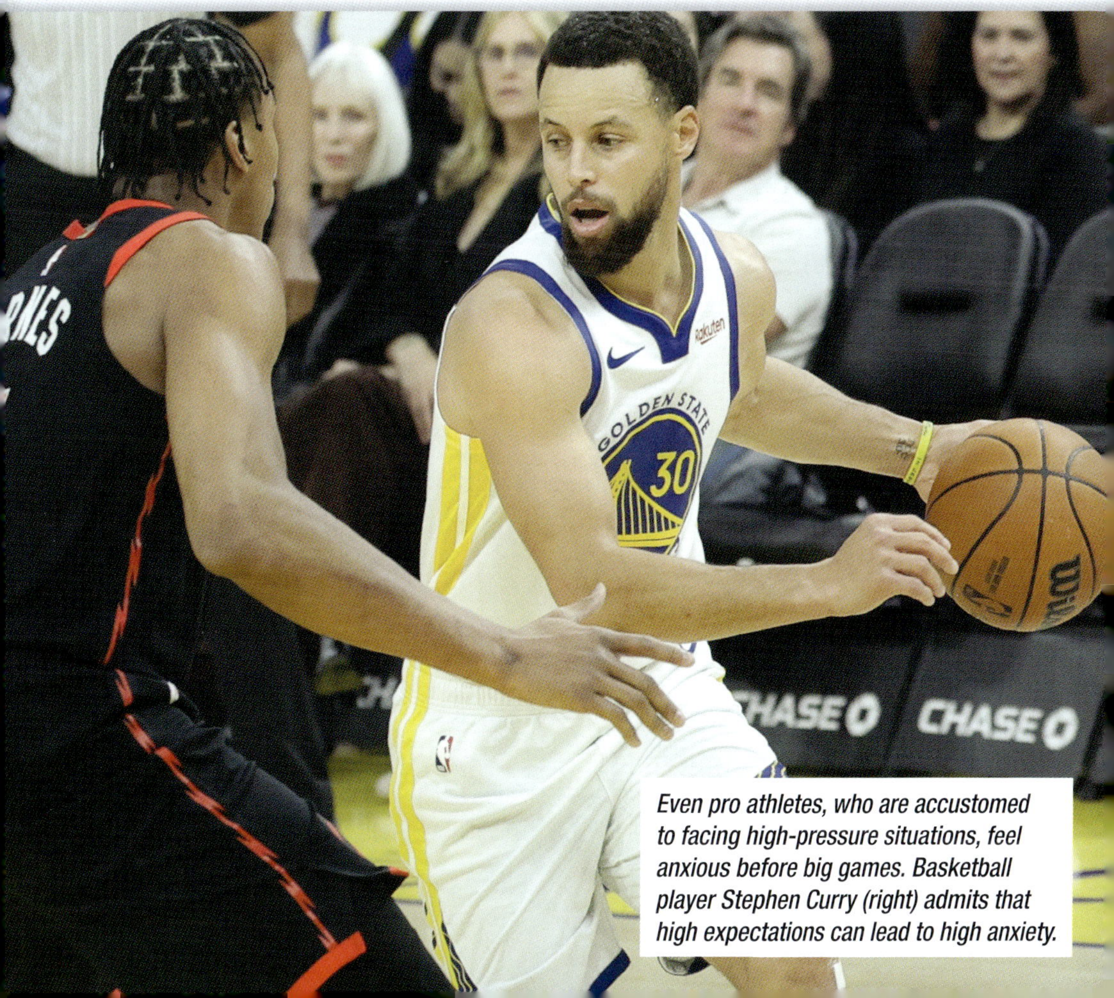

Even pro athletes, who are accustomed to facing high-pressure situations, feel anxious before big games. Basketball player Stephen Curry (right) admits that high expectations can lead to high anxiety.

Nick Hobson, a research psychologist and lecturer at the University of Toronto, has measured the effect of anxiety on brain power and performance. "Anxiety helps to hone our attention to what is directly in front of us, which is the brain's way of telling us that this thing (or person) is important and should be resolved or dealt with before moving on," says Hobson. In an experiment, Hobson gave a group of people difficult cognitive tasks to perform. He instructed the participants to remain calm and detached as they encountered errors—a suggestion meant to suppress any anxiety they might feel. Hobson then gave the group a second round of tasks. This time he told them to react to their errors as "an immersive experience where you really feel all the emotions."[7] This suggestion primed the subjects to accept the experience of anxiety.

> **"Anxiety helps to hone our attention to what is directly in front of us."[7]**
>
> —Nick Hobson, a researcher at the University of Toronto

When the participants were told to remain detached, they reported feeling less anxiety than when they were asked to accept their emotions. That was expected. But what was surprising is that when the participants were allowed to feel anxiety, they performed better on the tasks. "It's the negative emotions that matter most for driving our optimal performance,"[8] concludes Hobson.

Anxious feelings typically fade once a stressful moment has passed. The nervous energy a student feels before a test often disappears once they start answering questions. Stage fright often melts away once the performance begins and the actors begin speaking their lines. In such cases, anxiety actually helps people adapt to situations. It sharpens their focus, keeps them alert, and motivates them to prepare for the next stressful situation. Anxiety can be useful when it comes and goes at the right times.

When Anxiety Persists

For some people, however, anxiety does not fade away. Instead, it is a familiar companion. In some cases, the feelings of anxiety grow so strong that they begin to interfere with daily life. A person may worry constantly. Their sleep can be disrupted. Even simple tasks may feel overwhelming. At this point, anxiety stops being helpful and is considered harmful. The person may be suffering from GAD.

According to the *DSM-5-TR*, GAD is defined by excessive, uncontrollable worry occurring more days than not for at least six months about various events or activities. It also must be accompanied by at least three of six physical or cognitive symptoms. These include restlessness, fatigue, concentration issues, irritability, muscle tension, and sleep disturbance.

While some anxiety disorders, such as phobias, have a specific trigger or cause, GAD generally is a response to the pressures of everyday life—finances, jobs, school, friendships, and health. Since such concerns are commonplace, people suffering from GAD often do not realize that what they are experiencing is not normal stress. In addition, GAD's symptoms are physical rather than emotional, making it harder to identify their source. A person may not sleep well and feel fatigued, restless, and irritable during the day. They and those around them may dismiss these

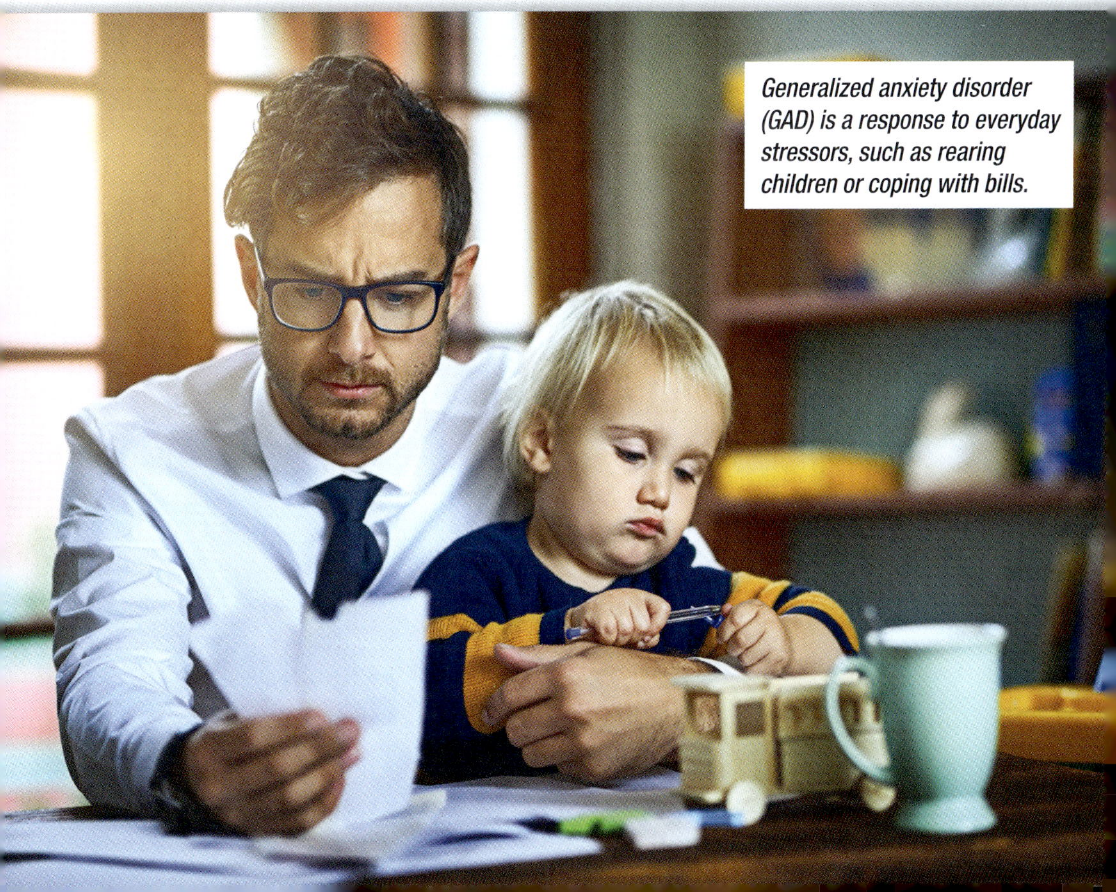

Generalized anxiety disorder (GAD) is a response to everyday stressors, such as rearing children or coping with bills.

How Anxiety Feels

Daneisha Carter had a panic attack when she was eighteen years old. Afterward, she did not feel the same as she had before. "I noticed I wasn't myself," she says. "I was angry or sad most of the time." Her anxious feelings persisted over time, meeting the criteria of GAD. She describes how GAD feels:

> In certain situations, like car rides, I would get super anxious, grabbing on the door handle because I was fearful something was going to happen to me. April 2022, I was at a fair with my cousin and brother, and there was a shootout. I have never been so scared in my life. It definitely amped up my anxiety. As time went on, it felt like my anxiety was getting worse and worse. I became very stressed out. I started losing focus on school, work, everyday tasks, and I had personal issues at home I was battling. My health even started to decline. Everything was happening all at once and I couldn't control it. I would cry myself to sleep every night. Wishing that all this pain could go away. I even became suicidal multiple times but never acted on it.

Daneisha Carter, "Finding the Light at the End of the Tunnel," Personal Stories, Anxiety and Depression Association of America, August 31, 2023. https://adaa.org.

symptoms as part of the sufferer's personality rather than a medical condition. As a result, GAD may go undiagnosed for years. "I used to suffer from an anxiety disorder," writes one Reddit user. "I feel like . . . the only problem was in my thinking."[9]

That is not to say that the symptoms of GAD are incidental or mild. They can be extremely intense. A mental health counselor named Lenibell Marak has struggled with GAD for years. Her eloquent description captures how overwhelming the disorder can feel:

> I have spent countless nights trapped in my own mind, where sleep feels like a distant memory and reality blurs into something unrecognizable. Anxiety doesn't just whisper—it screams. It fills my head with thoughts I never asked for, thoughts that claw at me, that make my heart race for no reason, that convince me something terrible is always waiting just around the corner.
>
> Drowning—that's the only way I can describe it. Sinking in a pool of thoughts so deep, so endless, that I can't see

the surface. The "what ifs" wrap around me like unseen currents, pulling me under. What if I'm not good enough? What if something terrible happens? What if I never get better? What if I die? The weight of it all presses down on me, and no matter how much I struggle, I can't seem to come up for air.

My anxiety doesn't rest. It lurks in the background, waiting for a quiet moment to strike. The thoughts feel so real, so vivid, that for a second, I almost believe them. That's the scariest part—how real it all feels.[10]

Other Anxiety Disorders

Anxiety can arise from many different sources, so it is not surprising that there are anxiety disorders in addition to GAD. These include social anxiety disorder, separation anxiety disorder, and phobias.

Social anxiety disorder is a persistent, intense fear of social situations. These feelings are different from the shyness or apprehension that people often feel in social settings. People with social anxiety disorder worry that they will be judged, scrutinized, or even humiliated by others. As a result, a person with social anxiety can feel intense fear about engaging in everyday activities, such as talking to strangers, eating or drinking around other people, or using public restrooms. Social anxiety sufferers often experience a heightened sense of self-consciousness, worrying that others will notice that they are anxious. While people who are shy can overcome their uncomfortable feelings, people with social anxiety disorder are paralyzed by them.

"My anxiety doesn't rest. It lurks in the background, waiting for a quiet moment to strike."[10]

—Lenibell Marak, mental health counselor

The fears of social anxiety are often accompanied by physical symptoms. These symptoms may include blushing, rapid heartbeat, trembling, perspiring, difficulty breathing normally, dizziness or lightheadedness, muscle tension, or an upset stomach or nausea. When people with social anxiety disorder exhibit one or

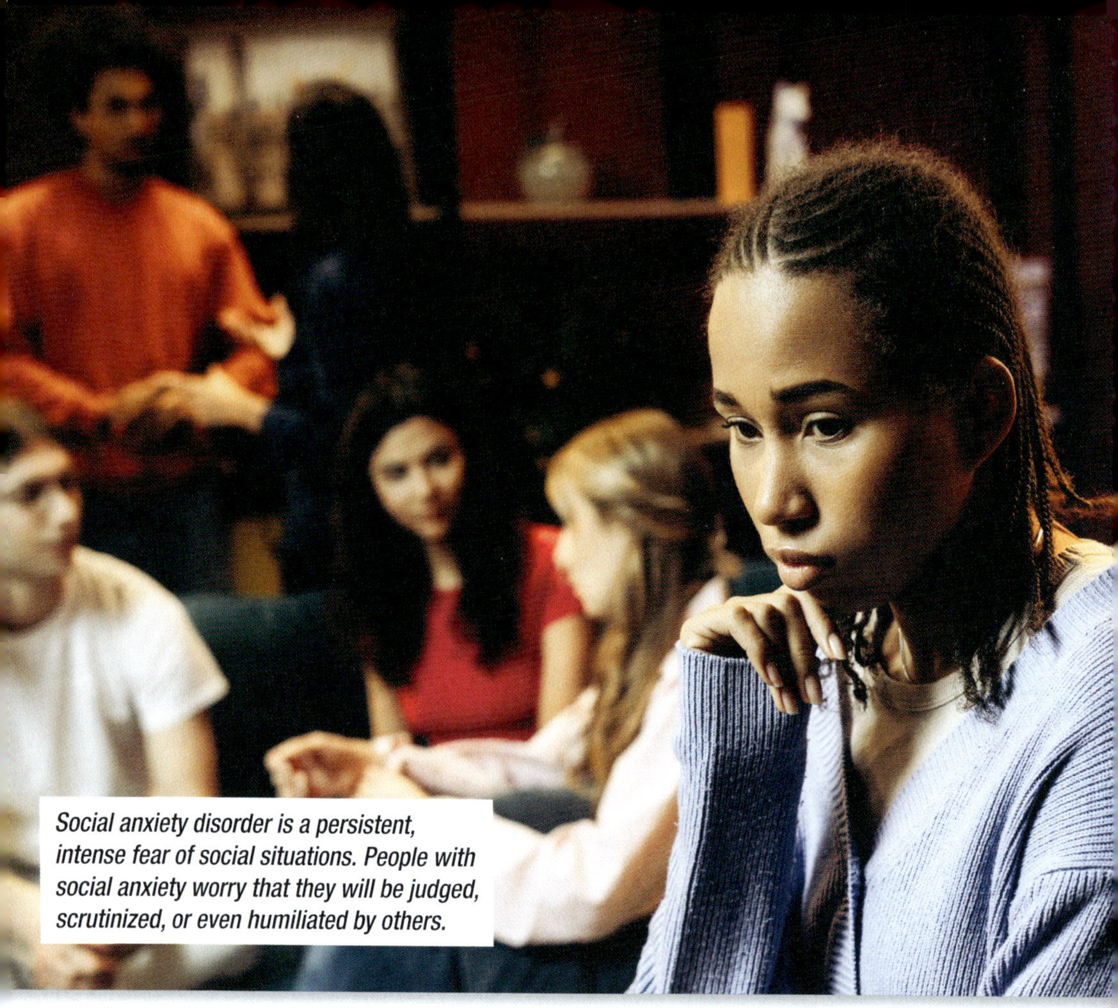

Social anxiety disorder is a persistent, intense fear of social situations. People with social anxiety worry that they will be judged, scrutinized, or even humiliated by others.

more of these physical symptoms, they can feel even more self-conscious, which in turn heightens their anxiety.

People suffering from social anxiety disorder often find that they are unable to control their worries and fears. As a result, they take steps to avoid the settings where their anxiety might surface. They stay away from situations such as meeting new people, eating in public, or even returning items to a store. In some cases, they might avoid school or work. When social anxiety becomes disruptive to everyday life for at least six months, it is diagnosed as a disorder.

Separation anxiety disorder is one of the most common anxiety disorders among children and adolescents. It is marked by an excessive fear or anxiety about being separated from attachment figures, typically a person's parents. Separation anxiety is normal in children ages eight to fourteen months, but generally it fades as children get older. It is considered an anxiety disorder when it involves an inappropriate intensity and lasts more than four weeks in older children and adults. In adults, the attachment figures shift from parents to spouses or romantic partners. Symptoms typically include an unwillingness to leave the home, physical complaints such as headaches and stomachaches, and extreme worry for loved ones' safety.

Anxiety can also be caused by what the *DSM-5-TR* calls specific phobia. Specific phobia is an intense, irrational, and persistent fear of a specific object, animal, situation, or activity that poses little to no actual danger. For example, some people are deathly afraid of all spiders, not just poisonous ones. Common phobias include the fear of flying, heights, certain animals, receiving an injection, and seeing blood. A phobia is considered an anxiety disorder when it persists for six months or more, causes a significant disruption of daily life, and is not better explained by the symptoms of another mental disorder.

Struggling with a Phobia

Specific phobia is an anxiety disorder characterized by fear or anxiety about the presence of a specific object or situation. In an online forum, a person about to undergo a dental procedure asked for support with their phobic fear of medical procedures involving hypodermic needles:

> I have a crown being put on in two weeks and I am so anxious and scared of the needle. I haven't had dental injections in years. I am crying sometimes. . . .
>
> My brain will not let it go. My brain keeps telling me I will be in excruciating pain, or I will move from the pain and make a huge gash into my gums, or the injection is going to distort my gums so bad my face and cheeks will be deformed. (Yes, I know this is just my stupid brain.)
>
> I am terrified of pain of the needle. I hate needles. I am terrified.
>
> I got Xanax (Alprazolam) to hopefully keep me calm so I don't flip out.
>
> I guess I am needing some reassurance that things will be okay. That it won't be excruciatingly painful.
>
> Help.

Plzdonthurtme, "Needle Fear—Terrified!," Dental Phobia Support, Dental Fear Central, April 9, 2025. www.dentalfearcentral.org.

Strength in Numbers

Anxiety disorders are extremely common. According to the NIMH, anxiety disorders affect more than 42 million adults each year. Among teens, the numbers are also high. Almost one in three—31.9 percent—of US adolescents ages thirteen to eighteen experience an anxiety disorder at some point in their lives. About 8.3 percent of teens report severe impairment from these disorders. Anxiety disorders are more common among female adolescents (38.0 percent) than male adolescents (26.1 percent).

The fact that so many Americans have an anxiety disorder can be a source of comfort to those who are experiencing one themselves. They realize that they are not alone and that millions of others are able to manage the condition and live satisfying lives. Anxiety is not a personal weakness. In small doses, it can be helpful for success. And if it is interfering with a person's life, it is treatable. Understanding what anxiety is—and what it is not—is the first step toward managing it.

CHAPTER TWO

Inside a Panic Attack

Ryan McCarney was a junior in college and a star baseball player with hopes of being drafted to play professional ball. Everything in his life seemed fine, but one night it all changed. "I was driving and I started to get short of breath," remembers McCarney. "My vision became blurry and almost shaky, and my adrenaline shot through the roof. I could feel myself getting ready to pass out." Afraid he might lose control of the car and injure himself or someone else, he acted quickly. "I pulled off the side of the road and got out," he recalls. He felt helpless. "I had to call my dad, who drove two hours to come get me and take me to the hospital." What happened next came as a complete shock. "They did the tests and they told me it was a panic attack. I was angry. I was a competitor, and there's no way my mind was doing this to me. But it was."[11]

"They told me it was a panic attack. I was angry. I was a competitor, and there's no way my mind was doing this to me. But it was."[11]

—Ryan McCarney, panic attack sufferer

The Common Roots of Panic Attacks

Panic attacks can often be traced back to something built deep into human biology known as the fight-or-flight response, which enabled early humans to survive the many dangers they faced. When the brain senses a threat—whether from a wild animal or simply a stressful situation—it sends a signal through the nervous system. The brain then floods the body with stress hormones, such as adrenaline and cortisol. As these hormones course through a person's body, the heart speeds up to pump blood to the muscles, the breathing quickens to bring in more oxygen, and the senses sharpen as the body prepares to either confront the danger (fight) or escape it (flight). The fight-or-flight response is automatic; a person does not choose to do it.

People today still experience the fight-or-flight response when they face a real danger. Individuals who have escaped from harrowing situations, such as a boating accident, a fire, or an airplane crash, often report having strength or stamina they did not know they possessed. This is the result of the surge of stress hormones the brain has released into their bloodstreams.

Sometimes, however, the fight-or-flight response is triggered by events that are not life-threatening. They may consist of no more than a confusing moment, a sudden worry, or even a misunderstanding. Nevertheless, the body's stress system, designed to protect against real threats, can activate even when no danger is present. A racing heart, tense muscles, or sudden dizziness may appear without warning, simply because the brain has sent a false alarm.

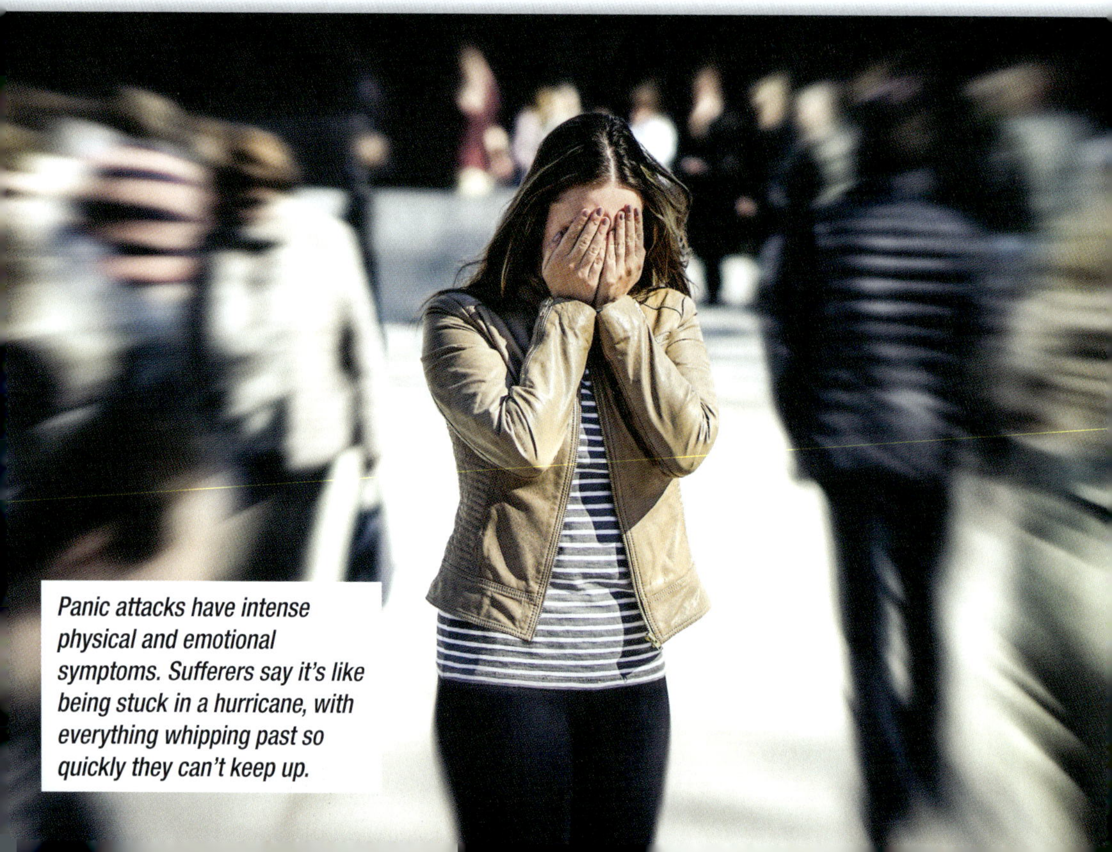

Panic attacks have intense physical and emotional symptoms. Sufferers say it's like being stuck in a hurricane, with everything whipping past so quickly they can't keep up.

"Anyone who has experienced a panic attack can probably agree with me when I say it's one of the worst feelings in the world," Annabeth Suchy wrote while she was a high school student in Ohio. "You feel like you're stuck in the middle of a hurricane. Everything is whipping past so quickly you can't keep up. You just shut down."[12]

Powerful Emotions and Physical Sensations

As powerful as a panic attack's physical symptoms can be, they are only part of the story—some would say the lesser part. A person having a panic attack can suffer emotional symptoms that dwarf the pain. These can include a sense of impending doom or danger, a feeling of unreality or detachment, or a fear of loss of control or death. For Brynn Burger, a panic attack produced certainty that her life was about to end. She describes it this way:

> It is 3:00 in the morning. I wake up from a dead sleep, sit straight up, and immediately know something is wrong. I am sweating, nauseous, and feel as if someone has dumped a bucket of ice water onto my chest. I feel it spill down my abdomen and through my arms and legs. My chest feels as though a giant's hand is squeezing it with the intention of taking my life.
>
> I feel like I am dying. . . .
>
> When I was in the middle of my panic attack, there was no person, no statistic, no test that could have convinced me that I wasn't living my last moments on earth. I felt like I was trapped in a nightmare.[13]

As in Burger's case, panic attacks usually come on quickly. Typically, they last between five and twenty minutes, with symptoms peaking within ten minutes. That is certainly long enough to convince someone they are seriously ill or even dying. Some people report panic attacks that last up to one hour. Typically, this is a series of shorter attacks with moments of high anxiety between them.

A Psychologist's First Panic Attack

Elaine Ryan was a practicing psychologist when she found herself facing a mental health crisis of her own. She recalls the experience:

> I had just finished a phone call late at night and felt what I could only describe as electricity travelling up through my legs. I wasn't too alarmed at this, as I had been experiencing similar sensations for about one month before, but not to this extent.
>
> Very quickly, I found it hard to breathe. My face was tingling, and the air was not getting in. I was suffocating. . . . I believed, without a doubt, that I was dying. I checked my pulse, and it was very faint. I was alone. After midnight, I ran to the apartment upstairs and started banging on the door that I needed help.
>
> I rang a friend who lived nearby, and she sent her husband around. . . . He drove me to the hospital. The journey was terrifying as I found breathing difficult, and my pulse felt weak. I was kept in the hospital until about 5 am while they did tests. Everything was okay. They said I might have had a panic attack and check in with my doctor during the day.

Elaine Ryan, "My First Panic Attack—a Psychologist's Personal Story of Recovery," Dr. Elaine Ryan, February 15, 2026. https://mytherapist.ie.

Although a panic attack may be brief, the intensity can leave a person feeling weak. Even after a person's body returns to normal, they may feel depleted of all their energy. Their legs may feel wobbly, as if they cannot support their weight. In a weakened state, the person might find their body continues to tremble. For a brief time, they might not be able to think clearly.

From Attack to Disorder

A panic attack can be a one-time event for some people, but it can become a recurrent problem for others. This is especially true when the first panic attack is so traumatic that people live in constant fear of having another. This heightened state of anxiety itself can contribute to more attacks. Some people have panic attacks once a month or even several times a week. When a person experiences a panic attack followed by at least one month of persistent worry about future attacks or their consequences (such as a fear of "going crazy"), they may have what is known as panic disorder.

According to the *DSM-5-TR*, to be diagnosed with panic disorder, a person's panic attack must include at least four of thirteen symptoms. These include: a pounding heart or accelerated heart rate; sweating; trembling or shaking; sensations of shortness of breath or smothering; feeling of choking; chest pain or discomfort; nausea or abdominal distress; feeling dizzy, unsteady, lightheaded, or faint; have feelings of unreality or detachment from oneself; fear of losing control or going crazy; fear of dying; numbness or tingling sensations; or chills or hot flashes. In addition, the panic attacks cannot be due to the effects of a substance, such as drugs or medication, or a general medical condition.

Finally, the sufferer must either worry about future attacks or exhibit significant behavior changes such as avoidance of situations that might trigger an attack, or both. Since these situations can be commonplace, such as being at school, at work, or in a car, avoiding them can significantly disrupt a person's daily life. "After a panic attack happens, the brain forms an association between its occurrence and the context of the episode (whereabouts, companions,

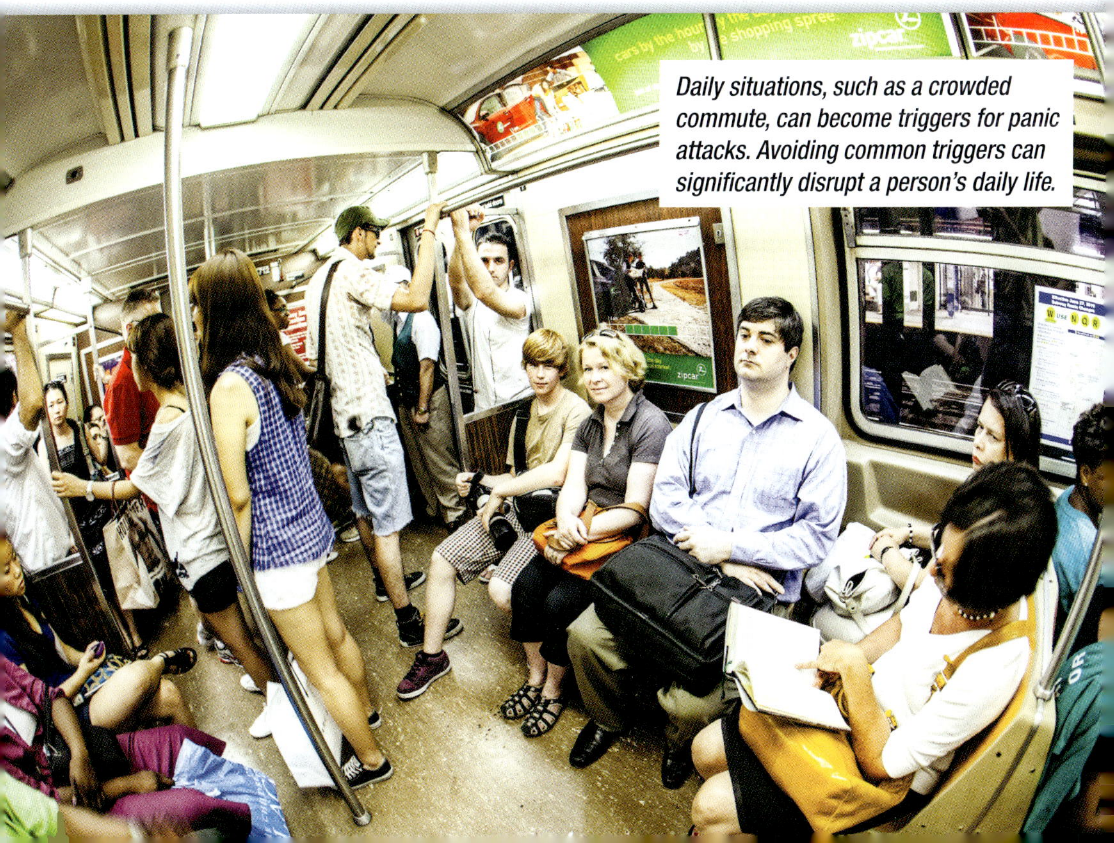

Daily situations, such as a crowded commute, can become triggers for panic attacks. Avoiding common triggers can significantly disrupt a person's daily life.

current activities, etc.)," explains Yasmina Rebani-Lee, cofounder of Mindriselife.org, an organization designed to help other people with anxiety. "This process leads to an automatic avoidance response to the site or context in which the panic attack occurred, whether it's a particular street, a certain comment or a specific activity."[14] Ironically, the very act of avoiding the situation reinforces the mental association, making the connection even stronger and leading to more avoidance. Sometimes simply thinking about the triggering event can cause another panic attack. The mind is trapped in a dangerous loop.

The Brain Against Itself

Carinne Deeds is one person who has been caught up in such a loop. "For the past few years, I've experienced increasingly frequent panic attacks and have developed a deep phobia of 'the next one,'" she says. "Unfortunately, the next one inevitably comes, perpetuating the painful cycle. This is the nature of panic disorder."[15]

Deeds describes panic disorder as a struggle between two parts of her brain—"Brain A and Brain B." She says that Brain A is her "normal" brain, the one that is capable of logic, reason, and the normal range of human emotions. Brain A recognizes that she is intelligent and is surrounded by people who love her. Brain B, she says, is the brain that takes over when she is having a panic attack: "Brain B is my fight-or-flight response. Brain B tells me I'm going 'crazy.' Brain B tells me I'm worthless. Brain B tells me that *this* panic attack will be the one that pushes me over the edge. Brain B tells me I have to leave the situation immediately, lest I lose all my friends and have to move back in with my parents. Brain B tells me that I am panic and panic is me."[16]

> **"Brain B is my fight-or-flight response. Brain B tells me I'm going 'crazy.' Brain B tells me I'm worthless."[16]**
>
> —Carinne Deeds, panic disorder sufferer

Deeds is emphatic that although Brain B strikes with the power of a hurricane, making her sweat, shake, vomit, and cry, its negative messages are not true. She says Brain B starts an internal struggle,

Carson Daly's Struggle with Panic Attacks

Carson Daly, cohost of NBC's ***TODAY*** show, has struggled with GAD and panic attacks for years. He has spoken publicly about his experiences. "You may think my life's perfect. I've got kids. I always look happy on TV," Daly says. "Things are not what they seem, and people need to know that's OK."

Daly recalls having a panic attack while on camera. "You think my right hand's in my pocket just being casual. . . . The truth is, in that moment, I was gripping the flesh of my upper right thigh because a wave of panic was coming through me, and I was so scared. I wanted to run off the stage because it's one of the symptoms of panic. I can't control my nervous system. Fight or flight kicks in. The threat is real, but there's nothing there."

Daly finally sought treatment for his anxiety. "Once you realize that other people have (GAD)—that it's an actual diagnosable thing, and there is a whole psychology and physiology behind it—you have context, and I think learning about all that, talking about it, exploring it has just ripped the veil."

Quoted in A. Pawlowski, "Carson Daly Recalls Wanting 'to Run Off the Stage' of 'The Voice' due to Panic Attack," *TODAY*, October 10, 2025. www.today.com.

but it never defeats her. She wants everyone with panic disorder to know they are not alone, and their situation is not hopeless.

Deeds says that she spent years suffering in silence. She never talked about her panic disorder because she was ashamed. She did not want to tell others that she had a voice in her head that was trying to convince her that she was crazy. Eventually, Deeds sought professional help. Slowly, this changed how she viewed her disorder. It took many hours of therapy, the support of friends and family, and a great deal of self-reflection, but she finally felt that she had won the war inside her head. Surviving panic disorder is now something she takes pride in.

Panic Disorder

Panic disorder is not as widespread as other anxiety disorders, but it still affects millions of adolescents. According to the NIMH, about 2.3 to 2.4 percent of adolescents (ages thirteen to eighteen) in the United States experience panic disorder in a given year. That translates to roughly 1.5 million teens annually. As with other anxiety disorders, there are gender differences in panic disorder. Panic disorder is more common among girls (2.6 percent)

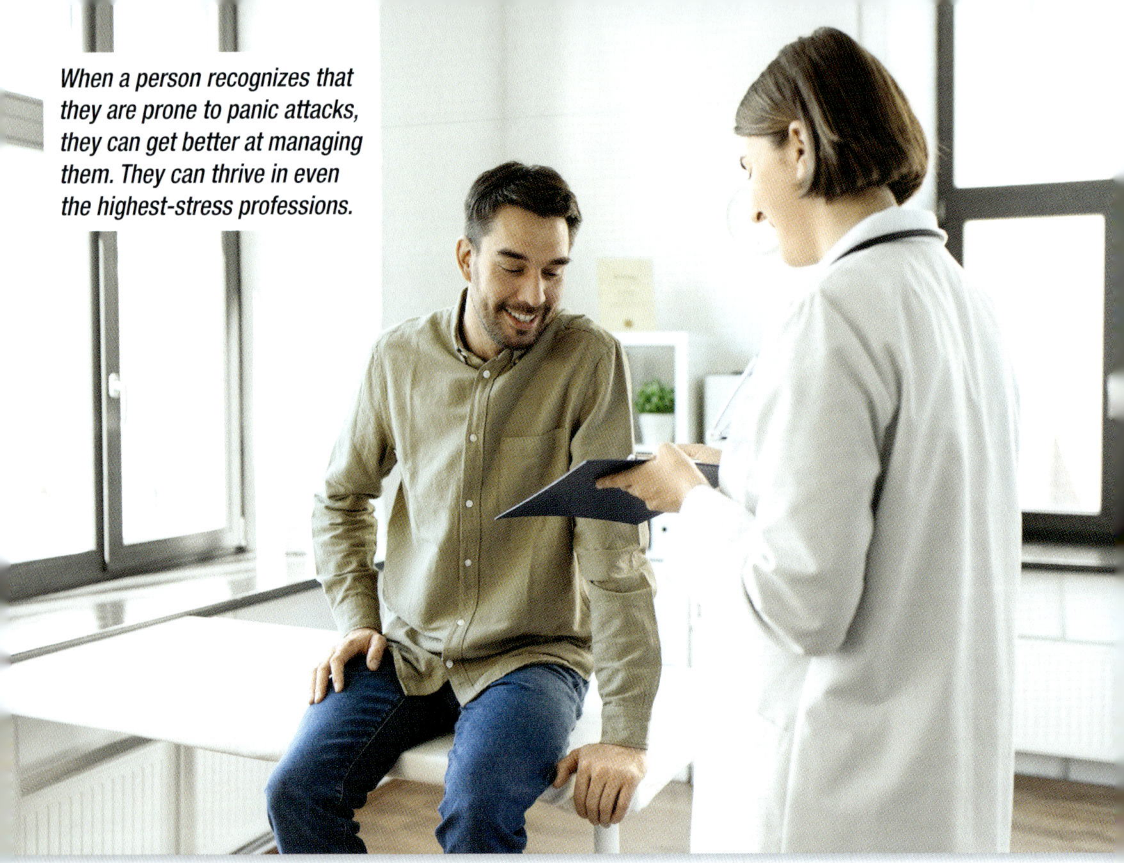

When a person recognizes that they are prone to panic attacks, they can get better at managing them. They can thrive in even the highest-stress professions.

than boys (2.0 percent). Among affected teens, about half report severe impairment, meaning the attacks interfere significantly with school, friendships, or daily life.

Once a person recognizes that they have panic attacks, they can become better at managing them. This is the case with Rebani-Lee. She remembers how she coped with panic attacks that came while she was a researcher, working on the twenty-second floor of a hospital. Her attacks would begin without any special cause or trigger. One time, she says, she was sitting in a chair, having a cup of tea and listening to the conversation of the people around her when she suddenly began to feel uncomfortable. She describes how the feelings surged:

> The feeling of discomfort grows exponentially in a matter of seconds; my pulse quickens, my heart races, my body shakes and my temperature rises. I know I have to do something. My breathing becomes shallow, I start sweat-

ing profusely and I begin to feel faint. Now I know I really must do something. I'm worried that I might be gasping for air very soon. To cope, I start looking around for exits, mentally tracing the various ways that will get me out of the building fast.

I note that the stairway is the best option as I certainly can't use the elevators and risk being stuck in one. Then, I remember the window. At that moment, I feel instant relief set in, knowing that if I need air, I can just open the window. My heart stops racing, and my breathing normalizes. In the clarity of my relief, I can now identify the episode as a panic attack.[17]

> **"I feel instant relief set in, knowing that if I need air, I can just open the window. My heart stops racing, and my breathing normalizes."[17]**
>
> —Yasmina Rebani-Lee, cofounder of Mindriselife.org

Panic attacks can feel bewildering, but understanding them can give people a sense of control. As the stories in this chapter show, the experience is intensely physical but can leave psychological scars. Recognizing the signs of a panic attack, acknowledging the fear, and learning how others have coped can break the cycle of confusion and shame. Whether a panic attack happens once or becomes a recurring challenge, it does not define a person. With knowledge, support, and practice, panic becomes something that can be anticipated, managed, and eventually eased.

CHAPTER THREE

Causes and Triggers

Panic attacks often arise from stressful situations or sensations—taking a big exam, participating in an important competition, or traveling to a new and unfamiliar place. The events that prompt panic attacks are known as triggers. They can vary widely from person to person, but they often follow recognizable patterns. By recognizing these patterns, people can often manage their reactions to them.

Although a panic attack may have a trigger, other anxiety disorders typically do not. They emerge from a combination of biological, psychological, and environmental factors. For example, some people feel anxiety more quickly than others because of their unique biology—the way their bodies react to stress. Other people carry memories or habits that shape how they interpret the world. Still others face daily pressures that gradually build until the body signals distress. Understanding these factors does not remove anxiety, but it can help people better manage it.

Biological Foundations

Some people are more sensitive to stress than others are. This sensitivity can be written in their genes. Anxiety often appears in multiple generations of a family. This suggests that certain inherited traits influence how the brain processes fear and uncertainty. "We've seen time and time again in studies of families that anxiety does run in families," says Anna Bauer, a psychiatric epidemiologist at UNC Health, an academic health network headquartered in

> "Anxiety does run in families. Children of parents who have a diagnosed anxiety disorder can be as much as seven times more likely to develop an anxious disorder themselves."[18]
>
> —Anna Bauer, a psychiatric epidemiologist at UNC Health

Chapel Hill, North Carolina. "Children of parents who have a diagnosed anxiety disorder can be as much as seven times more likely to develop an anxious disorder themselves."[18]

Brain chemistry also plays a significant role in anxiety. A person's neurotransmitters—the chemicals that allow neurons to communicate with each other throughout the body—help to regulate a person's mood. When neurotransmitters like serotonin and dopamine become unbalanced, a person can feel anxious.

Medical conditions can further complicate the picture. Thyroid disorders, asthma, chronic pain, and heart irregularities can produce sensations that cause anxiety. Even dehydration or low blood sugar can create shakiness or lightheadedness that contributes to anxiety.

Psychological Influences

Experiences and thought patterns also influence anxiety. Personal trauma, whether large or small, can leave a lasting impression. For example, if a person has experienced a traffic accident, the memory of it can feel very strong. If that person then sees a traffic accident on the road, it can heighten their anxiety because the sight reminds them of the traumatic event.

Similarly, a person who has endured bullying, loss, or family conflict may be especially vulnerable to anxiety. Even after the traumatic event has passed, the brain may remain alert, looking for anything that resembles the original threat. A crowded hallway, a raised voice, or a familiar smell can set off an internal alarm, even when the present moment is safe.

Sounds, places, smells, sights, people, events, and even dates can trigger emotions, including worry and fear. The emotions, in turn, can cause physical reactions, including muscle tension, increased heart rate, and shortness of breath—the classic symptoms of anxiety. For example, Christine Wolkin was swept off a

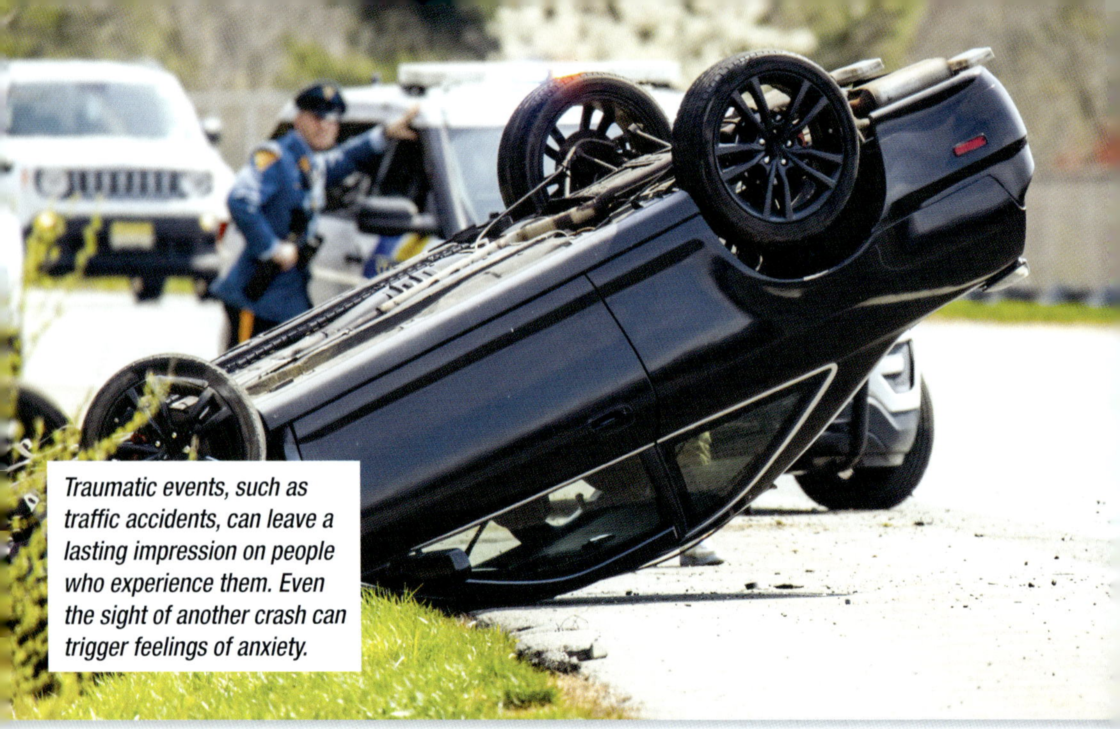

Traumatic events, such as traffic accidents, can leave a lasting impression on people who experience them. Even the sight of another crash can trigger feelings of anxiety.

rocky pier by a large wave when she was on vacation with her friends in Cancún, Mexico. She needed medical attention for an injury to her foot, but she was in a remote area where few people spoke English. The entire experience made her extremely anxious about traveling. A year later, she was overwhelmed with thoughts of impending doom when she traveled on a small boat, with her family, in the Caribbean. When she was driving home from the airport after that trip, the fears she experienced on the boat returned. "About an hour into my drive back to school, as my radio died and clouds began to roll in across the horizon, my heart started beating very quickly and my throat went dry," Wolkin remembers. "I started gasping for air, afraid my throat was closing and sped to the nearest exit."[19] The feelings passed, but it left an emotional scar that caused GAD. Wolkin recalls,

"Over the next several months I dealt with extremely uncomfortable and terrifying sensations when traveling by car."[20]

—Christine Wolkin, anxiety sufferer

> Over the next several months I dealt with extremely uncomfortable and terrifying sensations when traveling by car. I had no clue what was going on and I had no idea

what to tell people. Even the thought of getting into the car began to cause me excessive worry and physical sensations. As they got worse, I began to think I had a serious illness—maybe throat cancer—and started visiting my doctor, who told me it was just stress. I was given some medication—which I was terrified to use—and that was about it. I thought I was going crazy, I thought I was dying and had no one I could talk to that understood.[20]

Personality Traits

Anxiety can arise not only from traumatic events, such as Wolkin's experience of being injured while on vacation in a foreign country, but also from thoughts that a person carries inside. For example, some people feel they need to be perfect. The fear of making a mistake or disappointing others can turn ordinary tasks into sources of tension. When perfection becomes the expectation, anxiety often follows. The

Triggered by a Look

Bethany Chalmers suffers from anxiety and tardive dyskinesia (TD), a neurological movement disorder. Chalmers discusses some of the triggers that can heighten her anxiety.

> My anxiety can show up at any time and for seemingly any reason. When someone gives me a strange look, I instantly feel dread in the pit of my stomach. My muscles get tight as I wonder whether I did something wrong.
>
> Part of me understands that their weird glance likely has nothing to do with me; I just happened to be in their line of sight while they were lost in their own thoughts. Yet, the grip of anxiety and its never-ending *"what ifs"* often overshadow everything else. . . .
>
> Crowded places are one of my anxiety triggers. Being in a busy store can set off symptoms of severe anxiety—but I can't just leave. . . .
>
> As my anxiety grows, I become increasingly aware of the symptoms of my TD. Suddenly, I'm convinced my foot twitches and facial tics are getting worse and that everyone in the store is watching me.

Bethany Chalmers, "4 Strategies to Help Me Cope with Anxiety and Tardive Dyskinesia Together," Teva Pharmaceuticals, May 19, 2025. www.tevapharm.com.

mind begins to anticipate failure, even when success is likely. The fear of failure can create a worry that contributes to anxiety. "I have high expectations for myself but sometimes those expectations get in the way," Annabeth Suchy wrote while she was a high school student in Ohio. "It's like a never-ending argument inside my head. One side is constantly reminding me that I do not need to be perfect, while the other side is a constant repeat of 'but what if I *do*?' Eventually, the argument gets so loud it drowns everything else out."[21]

> **"It's like a never-ending argument inside my head. One side is constantly reminding me that I do not need to be perfect, while the other side is a constant repeat of 'but what if I *do*?'"[21]**
>
> —Annabeth Suchy, Ohio high school student

Fear of failure is one kind of negative thinking, but there are others that can also contribute to anxiety. Some people have recurring thoughts that something bad will happen or that everyone is judging them. These thoughts are not rooted in reality, but they can feel like facts. Once these thoughts become automatic, the brain responds to them as if they represent real danger. The result is a loop in which anxious thoughts create anxious feelings, and the anxious feelings reinforce the anxious thoughts. Once this mental loop is playing, an event that normally would not affect a person can resonate deeply, causing persistent anxiety.

Sometimes the negative thoughts feeding into anxiety have to do with a person's own health. Most people realize that individuals can get sick or may even have a serious physical ailment. That knowledge is cause for concern, but it usually does not cause overwhelming anxiety. However, when the person facing the medical problem already suffers from negative thoughts or has a biological sensitivity to anxiety, the diagnosis of an illness can make them feel worse. They might worry about a medical test or jump to conclusions about their condition. This can be terrifying and trigger anxiety.

Environmental Pressures

Not all of the factors that can trigger anxiety come from within a person. External events and pressures can also trigger an overwhelming fight-or-flight response. For example, a common trigger for teens and young adults is academic pressure. Many teens believe that a single misstep could harm their entire future. This belief is rarely accurate, but it can feel real. Suddenly, grades, deadlines, college applications, and extracurricular commitments take on exaggerated importance. These stresses accumulate until they feel overwhelming. When academic pressure builds without relief, anxiety becomes a natural response. The body reacts to the constant demand for performance by staying in a state of heightened alertness.

The same pattern exists when a person feels pressure not only from schoolwork but also from a job. A heavy workload, high pressure, and fears of making a mistake are often present in work situations. It is easy for people to ignore these pressures because they assume they are just a normal part of entering the workforce. As in an academic situation, the pressures can accumulate until they prompt a physical response from the body.

Even unpaid or volunteer work can contribute to anxiety. For example, family members may be caring for an elderly member of the family or someone who is seriously ill or dying. The demands

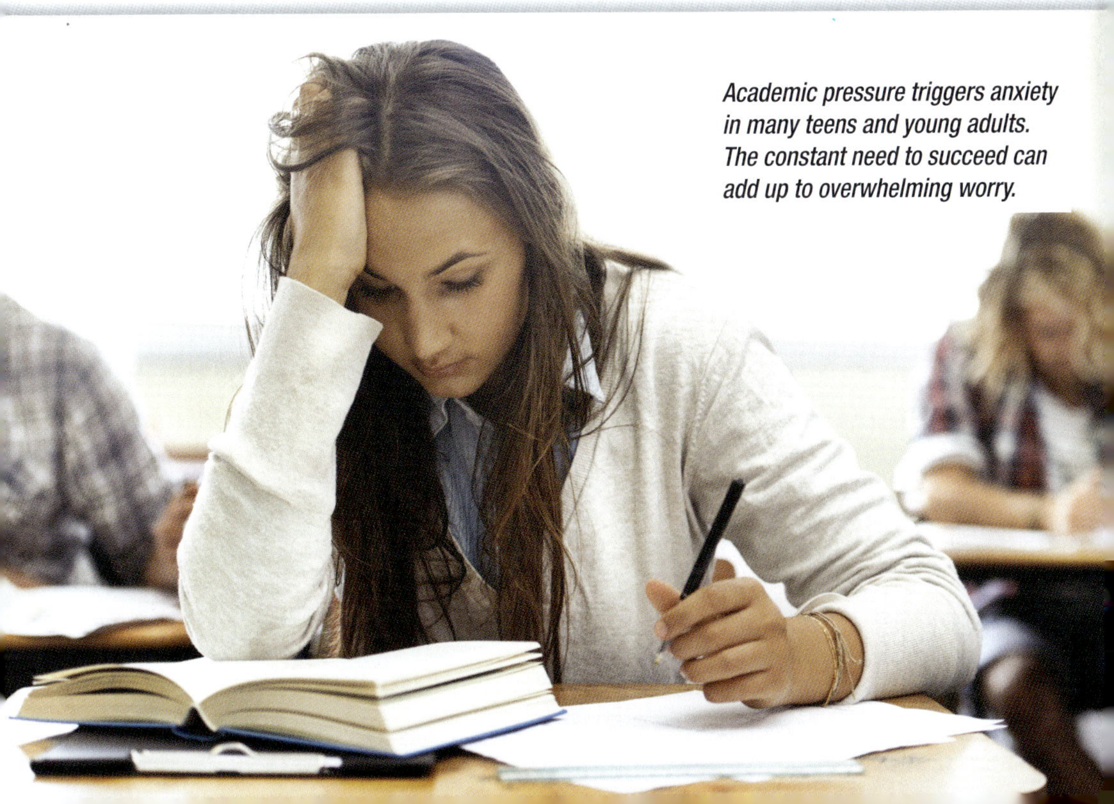

Academic pressure triggers anxiety in many teens and young adults. The constant need to succeed can add up to overwhelming worry.

can be high, and the fear of letting the family down can be enormous. Even house- or pet-sitting can invite pressures that create anxiety. Whenever a person feels pressure to meet a set of standards, the situation is ripe for anxiety.

Family dynamics can also contribute to anxiety. Arguments at home, financial stress, or responsibilities such as caring for siblings can create an environment where anxiety thrives. Even positive changes—moving to a new home or starting a new school—can produce stress simply because they disrupt familiar routines.

Social Media Pressures

Most environmental pressures have been afflicting people for decades or even centuries, but a new pressure has emerged in recent times: social media. Many social media users find that images

Everyday Strategies for Managing Anxiety

Paul McGregor, a speaker on mental well-being, has developed a four-step process for managing anxiety when he encounters triggers. He describes those steps:

1. Name it, don't fight it.
Instead of trying to "get rid" of anxiety, I acknowledge it. "I'm noticing I feel anxious right now." That small pause helps me separate who I am from what I'm feeling.

2. Calm the body first.
When anxiety kicks in, I take three slow breaths, drop my shoulders, and focus on the exhale. It reminds my body I'm safe, even if my mind hasn't caught up yet.

3. Lower the bar.
Anxiety thrives on perfectionism. So instead of doing everything perfectly, I aim for "good enough." Progress over perfection.

4. Talk before it builds.
When I feel it rising, I'll mention it to someone I trust like a colleague, friend, or family member. Every time, it loses a bit of its power.

If you're dealing with anxiety . . . right now, please know this:

You don't have to eliminate it to be great at what you do.

You just have to stop letting it drive the car.

Paul McGregor, "I Used to Think Anxiety at Work Meant Panic Attacks," LinkedIn, December 2025. www.linkedin.com/posts/pmcgregorcom_anxiety-work-activity-7381347018717306880-rl3L/.

of success, beauty, or popularity can make them feel inadequate, even though they may logically understand that the images they see are carefully curated or filtered. Because digital life never fully pauses, the stress it creates can feel unrelenting. Users of all ages are susceptible to this stress, but since teens tend to be more engaged with social media than adults and have not had time to develop strong defenses against social comparisons, they tend to experience more social media anxiety than anyone else. According to a survey by the Centers for Disease Control and Prevention, 50.4 percent of respondents ages twelve to seventeen reported spending four or more hours per day engaged with phone or computer screens. Of those, about one in four (27.1 percent) experienced anxiety during the previous two weeks. By comparison, only 12.3 percent of the participants with fewer than four hours of screen time reported having anxiety symptoms during the same period.

Comparisons are not the only pressures teens experience online. According to the Pew Research Center, 59 percent of US teens have experienced cyberbullying. This can take the form of offensive name-calling, hurtful rumors, and receiving unsolicited explicit images. Cyberbullying causes increased risk of anxiety, depression, and self-harm.

The Role of Self-Care

People often describe their anxiety as coming on without warning. This is the case because people sometimes do not realize that their habits or activities may have made their bodies vulnerable to an imbalance of hormones. A lack of self-care can put the nervous system into a precarious position. For example, a lack of sleep can intensify anxious feelings. A tired brain has a hard time regulating emotions and interpreting situations accurately. Small problems can feel enormous, and anxious thoughts can overwhelm a person.

What a person eats and drinks can also play a role in their mental health. Sometimes people consume coffee or energy drinks that are loaded with caffeine, a natural stimulant found in

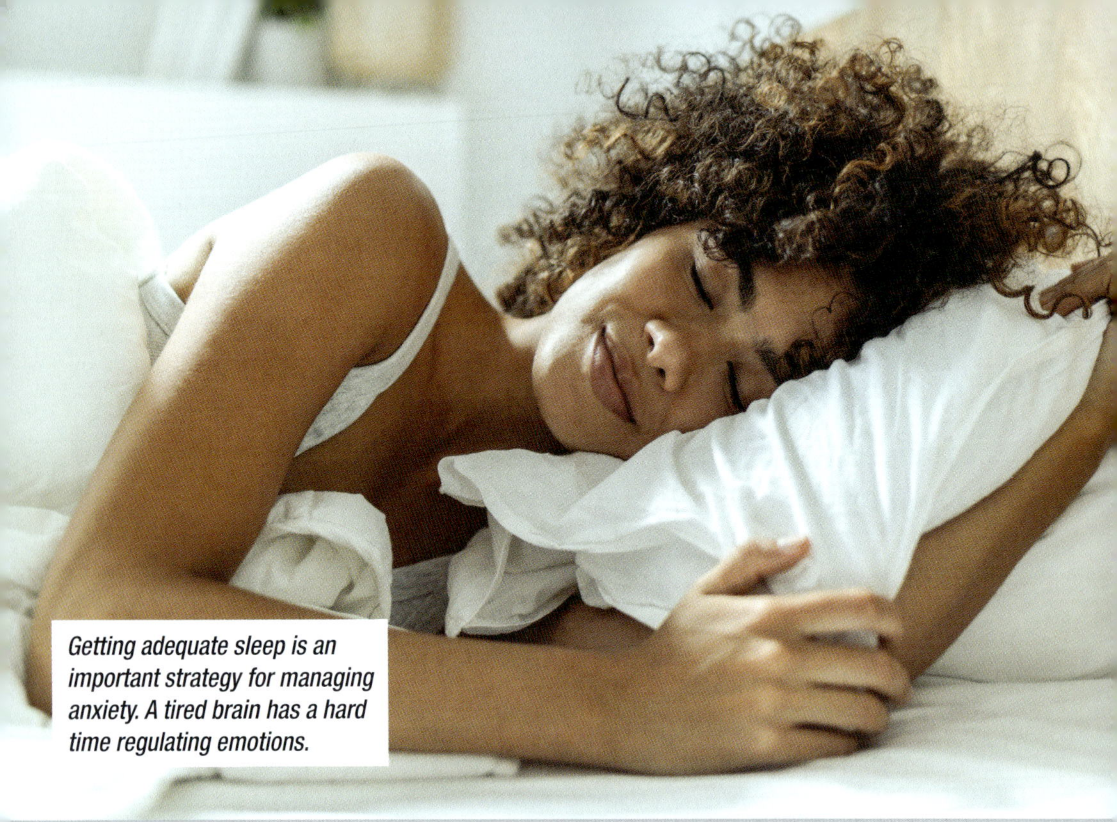

Getting adequate sleep is an important strategy for managing anxiety. A tired brain has a hard time regulating emotions.

coffee beans, tea leaves, cocoa pods, and kola nuts. Caffeine increases alertness, reduces fatigue, and speeds up bodily functions by blocking adenosine receptors in the brain. Normally, these receptors bind to a natural chemical known as adenosine throughout the day to eventually slow the heart rate and induce sleepiness. When a person needs to study or work late into the night, they may consume caffeine to fend off sleepiness. The combination of a rapid heart rate and a lack of sleep can worsen anxiety. Medications, including stimulants or decongestants, may also trigger anxiety by producing side effects that the brain interprets as dangerous.

Similarly, food—or the lack of it—can disrupt the body's normal functioning and, with it, the brain's resilience. For example, skipping meals can lead to low blood sugar (hypoglycemia). This condition can induce a fight-or-flight response, releasing the hormones adrenaline and cortisol into the bloodstream. Adrenaline increases heart rate and energy, while cortisol increases blood sugar to maintain alertness. This surge of energy and alertness when no danger is present can intensify anxiety. Too much food can also be a problem. Side effects of overeating, such as heartburn and stomach pain, may trigger anxious feelings. Eating too much or too little can cause sleeplessness as well, creating a combination of factors that set a person up for anxiety.

Anxiety, however, rarely arises from a single cause. A person may be facing work or academic pressure, suffer from a lack of sleep, have low blood sugar, and consume too much caffeine all at the same time. If a person has a genetic predisposition toward anxiety, the situation is even more precarious. When such known and unknown forces combine, anxiety can escalate quickly. Having a panic attack or suffering from an anxiety disorder is not a sign of personal failure. Rather, it is a response to real pressures—internal, external, and often both.

Identifying one's own triggers is an important step toward managing anxiety. When people are mindful of the details in their lives, they can often see patterns in the events contributing to their anxiety. Keeping a journal can help them uncover such patterns and gain a clearer sense of what is happening internally. When they can identify what sets off their symptoms, they gain power to change their response. Recognizing triggers does not mean eliminating stress completely, but it does make prevention possible. By learning to spot patterns early, people can take steps to reduce anxiety.

Getting Treatment

Many people who have an anxiety disorder describe it as the worst feeling they have ever had. The severity of anxiety disorders often makes people think that nothing can be done to prevent them or even make them less frequent. This is not the case. Anxiety is highly treatable. Statistics indicate that 80 to 90 percent of people who seek and follow treatment experience relief.

The three most common treatments used for anxiety are CBT, medication, and lifestyle adjustments. These approaches are considered the foundation of modern anxiety treatment. Each works in a different way, and many individuals benefit from using more than one.

Changing Conscious Thinking

CBT is one of the most effective treatments for anxiety. Its core idea is that certain psychological problems are caused by conscious thinking and behavior, not by any deep-seated, unconscious urges or feelings. By recognizing and modifying these patterns of thinking and behavior, the CBT patient can reduce or even eliminate their symptoms.

In CBT, individuals learn to identify automatic thoughts—often negative, exaggerated, or based on fear—that arise in stressful situations. Therapists help patients examine these thoughts and consider more balanced interpretations of them. For example, instead of assuming that a mistake will lead to disaster, patients learn to evaluate the situation more realistically. They realize that even if a mistake occurs, it will likely result in only a temporary setback. Over time, changes in negative thinking can reduce the intensity of events that provoke anxiety.

CBT also emphasizes behavioral strategies. For example, with the help of mental health professionals, individuals may face situ-

"CBT has helped me build up resilience, gain self-belief and enjoy life as much as I can."[22]

—Kasey, a CBT patient

ations they have been avoiding because they are afraid they will trigger anxiety. This process, known as an exposure exercise, is carefully planned and conducted in a controlled environment. By confronting fears in manageable steps, individuals learn that anxiety, while uncomfortable, is not dangerous and does not have to dictate their actions.

CBT is particularly effective in helping individuals manage triggers. By analyzing the thoughts and sensations that produce anxiety, patients learn how their minds and bodies respond to stressful situations. This awareness allows them to intervene sooner during the buildup to heightened anxiety. The intervention can reduce or even prevent an escalation of anxiety.

Millions of patients have benefited from CBT. Kasey is one of them. While in college she wrote, "CBT has helped me build up resilience, gain self-belief and enjoy life as much as I can." Her therapist, she says, "helped me to re-train my brain to help me deal with stressful situations and realise just how strong I am."[22]

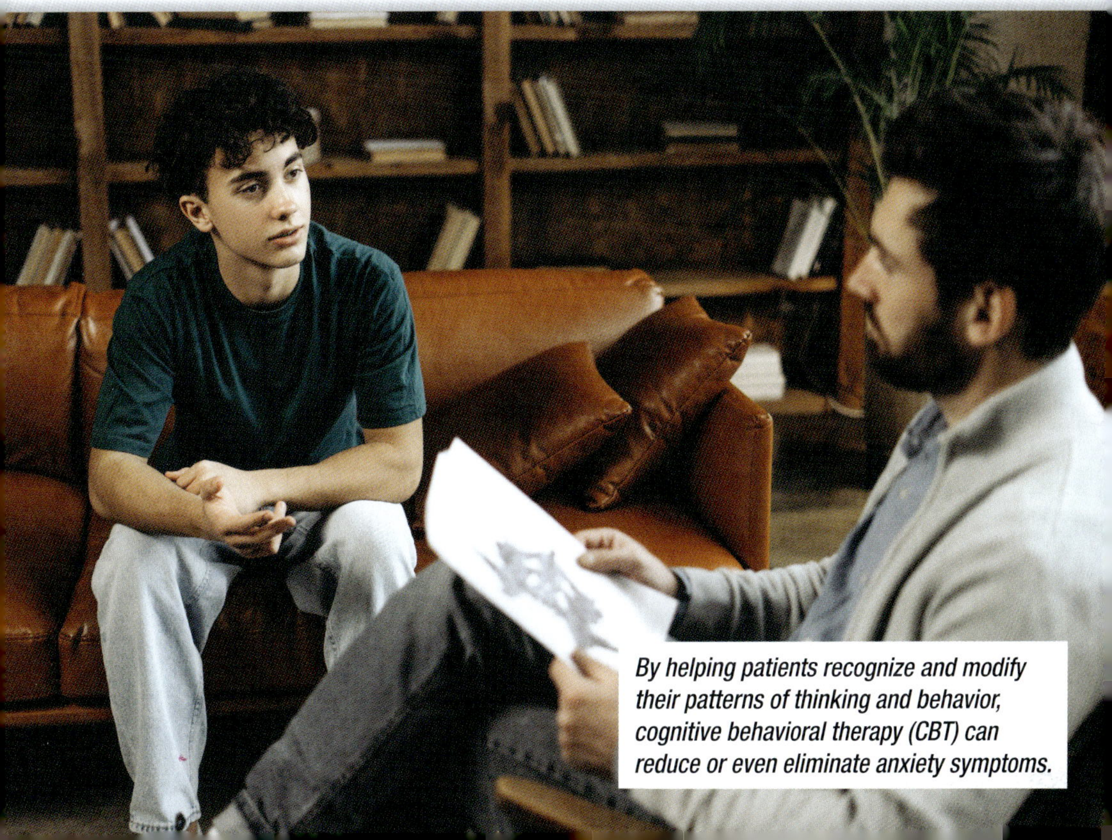

By helping patients recognize and modify their patterns of thinking and behavior, cognitive behavioral therapy (CBT) can reduce or even eliminate anxiety symptoms.

Acceptance and Commitment Therapy

Another therapy that uses conscious thoughts to manage anxiety is known as acceptance and commitment therapy (ACT). As with CBT, ACT patients work with mental health professionals to modify their thinking. ACT is different from CBT, however, because ACT encourages individuals to accept negative thoughts and feelings rather than challenging them or replacing them.

ACT has two main objectives. The first is for patients to accept the existence of unhelpful thoughts and feelings that cannot—and, in many cases, need not—be controlled. The second is for them to commit to living their lives according to their chosen values. By learning to coexist with uncomfortable emotions, individuals often find that anxiety loses some of its power.

Benefiting from CBT

Irshad, an IT professional, part-time blogger, and contributor to the online magazine Medium, credits CBT for helping him turn his life around. He writes,

> I never imagined I could break away from the never-ending cycle of bad ideas. For a long while, self-doubt and anxiety drove me into a mental prison. . . . I then discovered CBT, and it transformed everything. . . .
>
> My therapist emphasized that CBT is about understanding the relationship between our ideas, feelings, and actions. Although this seemed easy, it opened my eyes to how I had been locked in negative thought habits. . . .
>
> CBT taught me to become more conscious of my own thinking. I learnt that I had the power to shape my ideas. I discovered I don't have to believe every lousy notion that pops into my thoughts. With practice, I can pick a new route. . . .
>
> I won't state that CBT addressed all my difficulties. I still have bad days. Sometimes, my old thoughts want to come back in. But I now have the tools to manage them. I feel more in control of my thinking and my life.

Aamil_MS, "How Cognitive Behavioral Therapy (CBT) Transformed My Mental Health," Medium, February 7, 2025. https://medium.com.

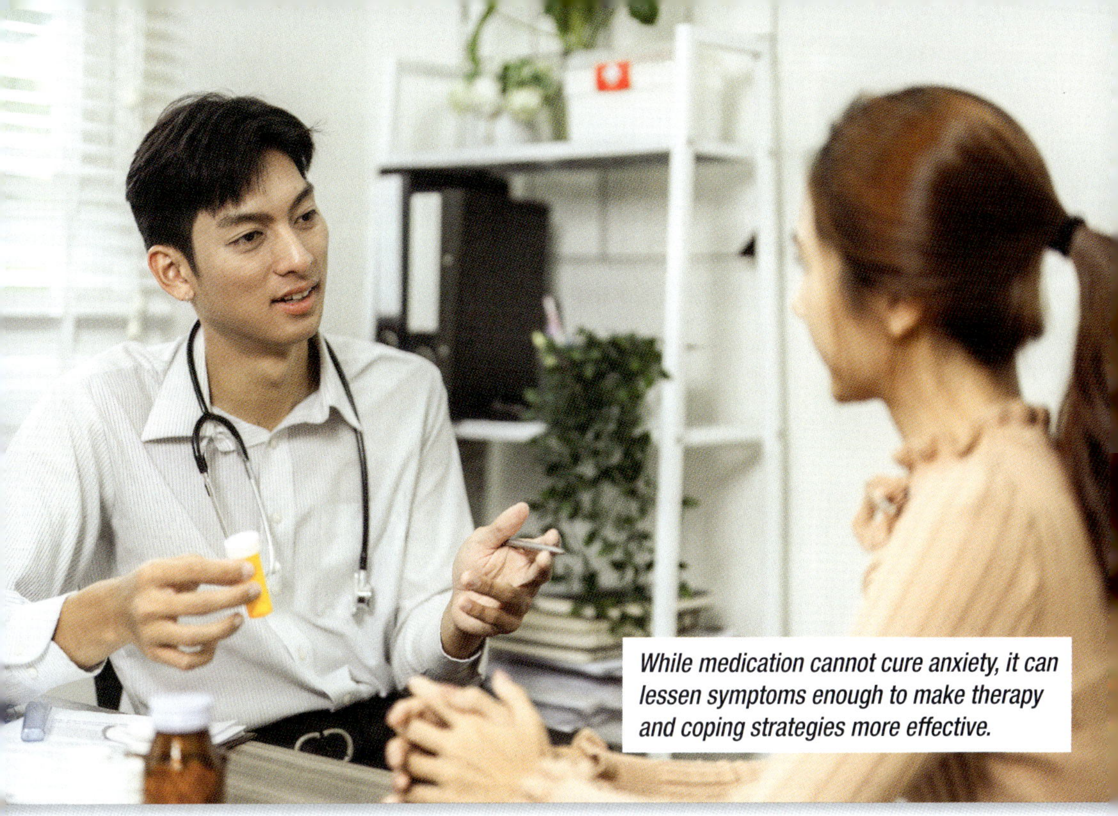

While medication cannot cure anxiety, it can lessen symptoms enough to make therapy and coping strategies more effective.

Medication

Although CBT and ACT can be effective, it takes time to master the techniques. In the meantime, a doctor or psychiatrist may prescribe medication to decrease anxiety. Medication is not a cure, but it can lessen symptoms enough to make therapy and coping strategies more effective. Finding the right medication can take time. Doctors often adjust dosages or try different medications before settling on the most effective plan.

Different medications work in different ways. Some help regulate the brain's response to stress. Selective serotonin reuptake inhibitors (SSRIs) increase serotonin levels to improve mood and lower long-term anxiety. Common prescription options include sertraline (Zoloft) and fluoxetine (Prozac).

Another class of anxiety medications are serotonin-norepinephrine reuptake inhibitors (SNRIs). These regulate not only serotonin but also norepinephrine, a chemical that functions as both a neurotransmitter in the brain and a hormone in the body. Norepinephrine is primarily responsible for the fight-or-flight stress response, and SNRIs help to manage it. Examples of SNRIs include venlafaxine (Effexor) and duloxetine (Cymbalta). SNRIs sometimes help patients who do not benefit from SSRIs. A Reddit user says he was reluctant to use medication for his anxiety, but in the end, he was glad he did. He writes,

> Over time this new psychiatrist kept urging me to get on SSRIs or SNRIs. I told him that I have tried them on and off for a decade plus with little to no results. . . . And after working with me for some months he finally recommended [an SNRI] drug called duloxetine. . . .
>
> The first 2 or 3 weeks starting the medication were expectedly uncomfortable. And I'm going to be honest with you, when you have severe anxiety these anti depressants are going to make you feel strange for a couple weeks. But over time I subtly am starting to feel better. It's taken about 6 weeks for them to kick in, and some of the side effects still linger, but it's manageable. I don't feel numb, I don't feel like a zombie or a different person. If anything, I feel more like myself. It's subtle. I still have depression, and anxiety and panic attacks. But I just feel generally more stable, feel like I can handle things more, my mood swings are less violent and frequent.[23]

Another approach using medications is to balance serotonin and dopamine to reduce worry and anxiety. A medication that does this is buspirone (Buspar). It works by affecting serotonin receptors in the brain.

Instead of affecting a person's moods directly, some medications are aimed at moderating the physical symptoms of stress. Effective medications for managing physical stress symptoms include the beta-blockers propranolol (Inderal) and atenolol (Tenormin). They block receptors in the brain, preventing them from producing physiological responses such as rapid heart rate or

> "It's taken about 6 weeks for [the medications] to kick in, and some of the side effects still linger, but it's manageable. I don't feel numb, I don't feel like a zombie or a different person. If anything, I feel more like myself."[23]
>
> —A Reddit user

shaking. By managing physical stress symptoms, beta-blockers prevent the brain from overreacting to stressful situations.

When a patient is suffering from severe anxiety and needs immediate help, a doctor may prescribe a class of medications known as benzodiazepines. These medications include alprazolam (Xanax), diazepam (Valium), and lorazepam (Ativan). They provide fast-acting relief for acute anxiety. However, they present a high risk of dependence, so they generally are reserved for short-term use.

Medication is often most helpful when anxiety is severe, persistent, or interfering with daily functioning. Medications can provide stability, allowing individuals to participate more fully in therapy or make lifestyle changes that support long-term recovery. While beneficial, medications are also known to have side effects. Patients who use medication must be willing to communicate any side effects or concerns to their health care provider.

Lifestyle Changes

Many medications act directly on the brain to balance its chemistry. However, a person can also make lifestyle changes that will help to regulate the nervous system. These lifestyle changes are low cost and relatively easy to make. They are not quick fixes, but over time they can make a person feel more balanced and better equipped to handle stress.

The foods and beverages a person consumes can affect the brain. Eating regular meals, staying hydrated, and limiting stimulants such as caffeine can reduce physical sensations that mimic or intensify anxiety. Because caffeine is a common trigger, many individuals find that reducing consumption of coffee, tea, and energy drinks leads to noticeable improvements.

Sleep is one of the most important factors in building resilience and preventing anxiety. Irregular sleep patterns, late-night screen use, and chronic fatigue can heighten anxiety and make symptoms more likely. Establishing consistent sleep routines can significantly improve emotional stability. One key to getting a good night's sleep is to create a calm bedtime environment. It begins with keeping the sleeping space cool (60°F to 67°F). The space should also be dark and quiet. Individuals can use blackout curtains to keep outdoor light from seeping in, and they should remove digital devices with glowing screens.

If the environment is not quiet, some people use earplugs or noise-canceling headphones to block out disruptions. Others invest in a white noise machine. This device masks disturbances by emitting consistent, soothing, and ambient sounds. "White noise can be a powerful sleep aid, especially for Gen Z, who are often immersed in a digital environment where silence is scarce,"[24] says Chelsea Perry, a board-certified sleep medicine specialist. A 2024 survey by Talker Research found that 49 percent of Gen Z respondents said they rely on white noise to sleep—the highest of any generation surveyed.

> **"White noise can be a powerful sleep aid, especially for Gen Z, who are often immersed in a digital environment where silence is scarce."[24]**
>
> —Chelsea Perry, a board-certified sleep medicine specialist

A person's routine before bedtime can be as important as the environment. Experts recommend creating a consistent thirty- to sixty-minute period that is tech-free and relaxing to signal to the body that it is time to sleep. Another signal to the body can be sent by dimming artificial lights. This tells the brain that darkness is approaching, prompting it to release the sleep-inducing hormone melatonin.

While rest is important for the brain, so is activity. Regular physical activity helps regulate stress hormones and release tension. Exercise does not need to be intense. Walking, stretching, dancing, or recreational sports can all contribute to improved mood and reduced anxiety. The body and the mind can also work together to reduce anxiety through exercises known as mindfulness practices. These can include meditation, yoga, or deep breathing. These techniques calm the body's stress response. By

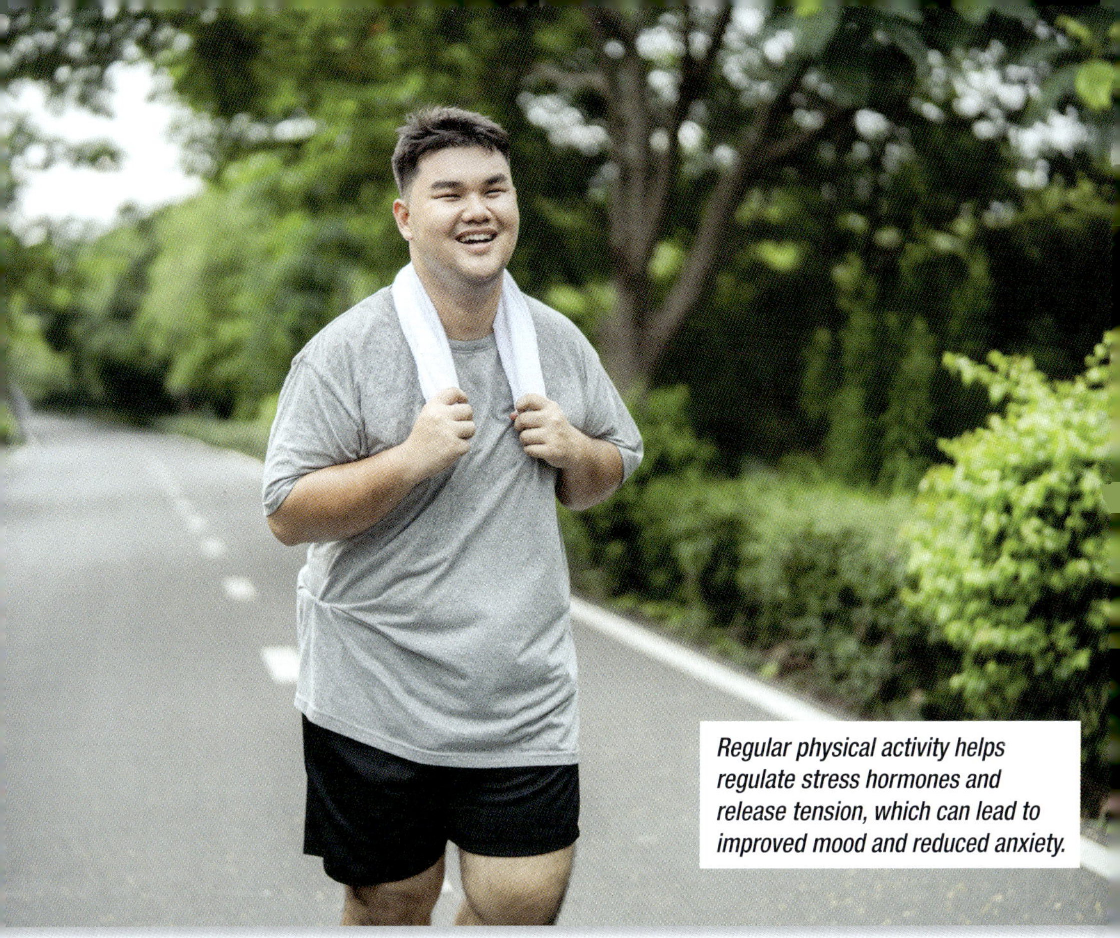

Regular physical activity helps regulate stress hormones and release tension, which can lead to improved mood and reduced anxiety.

focusing attention on the present moment—thoughts, feelings, body, and surroundings—a person can reduce concerns about the future, which are the cause of anxiety.

Emerging Therapies

Although CBT, ACT, medication, and lifestyle changes remain the core of anxiety treatment, new approaches continue to expand the range of options available. These emerging therapies reflect advances in psychology, technology, and neuroscience. They offer new options for people who need alternatives or supplemental support.

Mobile phones hold great potential for treating anxiety. More than 6.5 billion people around the world, including 95 percent of US teens (ages thirteen to seventeen) have access to a mobile phone. Users keep their phones within reach and check them many times a day. Treatment delivered via a mobile phone app can be accessed anytime and anywhere. Users can employ the app as needed throughout the day to prevent the onset or escalation of symptoms in moments of need. In addition, the systems can grow "smarter" by applying machine learning algorithms to data from the app's automatic monitoring systems or the user's inputs. This allows treatment content to be regularly updated and personalized to the needs of the user.

Mobile phones, tablets, and computers can also be used for remote therapy, or teletherapy. For example, a person with anxiety can video chat with a therapist. Meeting with a therapist online can reduce barriers related to transportation, scheduling, or geographic location.

Sometimes talking with peers can help a person manage anxiety. Online support groups and forums provide spaces where individuals can share experiences, ask questions, and feel less isolated. While these communities are not a substitute for professional care, they can complement treatment by offering connection and understanding.

A 2024 study published in the journal *World Psychiatry* found that nearly half (48 percent) of the apps used to manage anxiety were based on CBT principles. About 21 percent of the apps were based on mindfulness, and 10 percent used ACT techniques.

A Medication Success Story

A Reddit user talks on the platform about how she has suffered from anxiety her whole life. Writing for a Reddit community dedicated to anxiety, she says that Prozac has been beneficial for her:

> I have had severe anxiety since childhood, and I literally don't remember [when] there was [a] time I was calm and happy. I always was anxious, terrified, depressed and scared of everything, but, man, Prozac changed my life. I was terrified to take meds for my unending anxiety, but I eventually did [take] Prozac and I'm living my best life right now and I didn't know people experience life in a calming, fun way.

Desperate-Gift-7163, "Prozac Changed My Life," Anxiety subreddit, Reddit, February 2024. www.reddit.com/r/Anxiety/comments/1bosuti/prozac_changed_my_life/.

Some of the apps, about 14 percent, offered human guidance to the user. A small number, 5 percent, replaced human therapists with chatbots. About a third of the apps (34 percent) featured technology that monitored the user's moods. These tools make coping strategies more accessible, especially for individuals who may not have regular access to in-person therapy.

Virtual Reality Exposure

Virtual reality (VR) technology has been shown to be effective in the treatment of anxiety. In VR therapy, patients wear a headset that presents a realistic digital environment of sights and sounds. Therapists are able to control the virtual environments so their patients can gradually face their fears. VR exposure offers a level of safety that can be difficult to achieve in real-world settings. It also allows individuals to progress at their own pace, with immediate support from a therapist.

Challenges in Accessing Treatment

Though effective anxiety treatments exist, many individuals face obstacles when trying to access them. Some of these challenges lie within the person struggling with anxiety. Some individuals worry that seeking treatment will be seen as a sign of weakness or instability. This belief can keep them from seeking treatment, even when symptoms are severe.

Even when individuals recognize that anxiety is a legitimate health condition, they may be uncertain about how to seek treatment. Finding the right therapist, the right medication, or the right combination of strategies often involves trial and error. This process can be frustrating, especially when progress feels slow, but adjustments are a normal part of treatment.

Sometimes cost is a barrier to seeking help. Therapy can be expensive, and not all communities have an adequate number of mental health providers. Transportation, scheduling conflicts, and long waiting lists can also make treatment difficult to obtain.

Digital tools and teletherapy have helped address some of these barriers, but gaps remain.

Despite these challenges, millions of people are able to find and receive treatment. Nevertheless, treatment for anxiety and panic attacks is not a quick or simple process. It requires time, effort, and patience. Some individuals respond quickly to therapy or medication, while others need to try several approaches before finding relief. Progress often comes in small steps rather than dramatic breakthroughs, but these small steps can lead to a journey that improves their lives. The skills they learn do not eliminate anxiety entirely, but they make it possible to navigate stress, manage triggers, and prevent panic from taking over, laying the groundwork for long-term stability.

Living with Anxiety and Panic Attacks

Tanya Guschina is a professional illustrator who has lived with obsessive-compulsive disorder (OCD) and anxiety since childhood. "As a child, I went to bed fully dressed with my school backpack strapped on, convinced it would guarantee good grades," she remembers. "In college, I sometimes returned home just to put on my sneakers in the 'correct' order—right first, then left—because my brain insisted on it." She did not seek help for many years. "I hid my habits, even from family, thinking no one could understand." Eventually, however, she sought treatment. She tried a couple of different antidepressant medications, but with time she learned that practicing her art was the best way to manage her anxiety:

> Through all of this, I discovered that art is more than work; it's survival. Painting and illustrating became ways to structure the chaos in my head, give my anxiety a voice, and create spaces where I could breathe. It's in this space—my "Mental Room"—where my fears, obsessions, and creativity coexist, and where I can transform struggle into something others might recognize, relate to, and maybe even find hope in. . . .
>
> In this room, I write and illustrate one forbidden truth each day. The pressure and chaos of the pencil on paper let me trace the tension inside me, turning anxiety into something tangible. Some days the lines are frantic, jagged, almost

violent; other days they are soft, deliberate, revealing a rare moment of calm. It's a dialogue with myself—a way to understand what I cannot always speak aloud.

For me, art is not just a profession; it is my lifeline, my witness, and my proof that life with OCD and anxiety can still be rich, meaningful, and, at times, even beautiful.[25]

Managing Anxiety with Creativity

Guschina's method of managing anxiety is not unique to her. Martha Beck, an author and life coach (a professional mentor who helps clients improve their overall well-being), has built a therapy around tapping into a person's creativity. She points to research that has shown that the part of the brain used for analytical thinking and speech—the left hemisphere—is the same part of the brain that increases anxiety. As a result, logical thinking can make it harder to find relief. "All animals have fear responses when they're in danger," writes Beck. "But because of our fancy powers of speech and imagination, we humans can keep that fear response elevated indefinitely, whether we're in danger or not. In fact, the more left-brain dominant our society becomes, the more we as individuals receive messages to keep our angst spiraling up and up and up and *up* into ever-higher levels of anxiety."[26]

> **"Painting and illustrating became ways to structure the chaos in my head, give my anxiety a voice, and create spaces where I could breathe. . . . Art is more than work; it's survival."[25]**
>
> —Tanya Guschina, professional illustrator

In her book *Beyond Anxiety*, Beck discusses how she uses creativity to manage her own anxiety. "I was particularly intrigued by the evidence that shows a kind of toggle effect between anxiety and creativity: when one side is up and running, the other seems to go silent," she writes. "I began to play with something I call 'the art of calm,' because it was all about using creativity to calm my anxiety."[27]

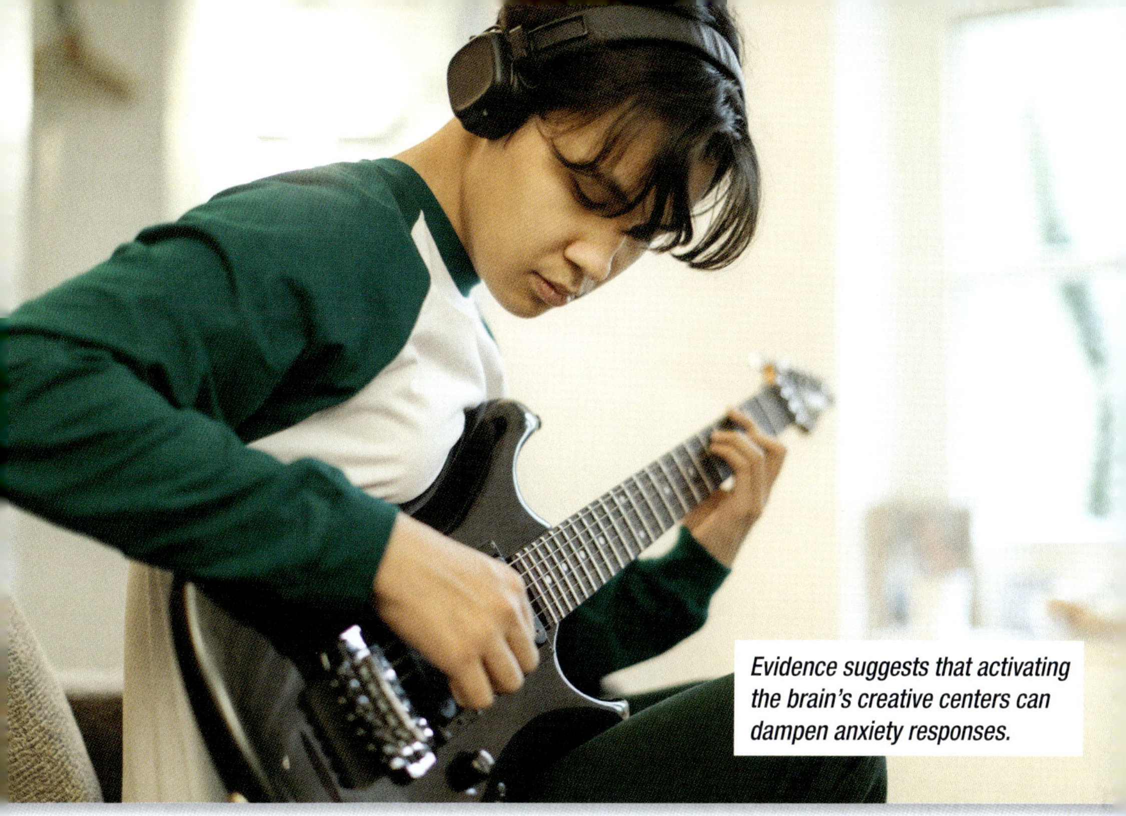

Evidence suggests that activating the brain's creative centers can dampen anxiety responses.

Beck argues that anxiety cannot be ended; it can only be replaced. "Even if we can relax our highly developed anxiety circuits, they collide with many forces (inside and outside our brains) that rev them back up—unless we fill the space where anxiety used to be."[28] In her therapy, Beck uses creativity to fill that space, providing her clients with exercises to engage the creative parts of their brains.

The Power of Journaling

Although the part of the brain involved with speech can create anxious thoughts and scenarios, some people are able to use that part of the brain to calm their anxiety. For anxiety sufferer Lenibell Marak, journaling became a way to manage her anxiety. She recounts how important writing became to her:

> I felt stuck, trapped in a body I didn't love, in a mind that didn't feel like mine. . . But something in me refused to let go. A tiny flicker of hope, a whisper beneath all the noise, that kept me holding on. . . .

> So, I took a step. I started therapy and I saw a psychiatrist. . . . I began changing small things. . . . Journaling saved me—I wrote [in my journal] when I was suffering, in the exact moment of my pain. These words are raw, unfiltered, real. Writing became my escape, my way of untangling the chaos. And slowly, I started seeing myself in those pages—the real me, not just the anxiety.[29]

"Writing became my escape, my way of untangling the chaos. And slowly, I started seeing myself in those pages—the real me, not just the anxiety."[29]

—Lenibell Marak, mental health counselor

Marak went on to earn a master's degree in clinical psychology and serve as a mental health counselor at a high school, hospital, and in her own private practice. "If there's one thing I've learned, it's that I'm still here," she writes. "Despite the drowning thoughts, the what-ifs, the sleepless nights, the fear, the anger, the tears—I'm still here. Anxiety is loud, but I am learning to find quiet."[30]

Coping with Fear

Abby Paradis is a writer and editor whose daughter suffers from a fear of swallowing food because she once choked on a handful of bite-sized cookies. Paradis, who also suffers from anxiety, has helped her daughter find good counselors and learn important calming techniques. More than a year after the choking incident, Paradis believes her daughter is making progress in managing her anxiety. She writes:

> I've witnessed an interesting shift. Radical honesty may be a useful tool. She names her anxiety. She asks for help in meeting her unique needs in those moments. She stands up in the middle of dinner, grabs an ice pack, drapes it across her neck, and sits, saying, "Wow, anxiety is so overwhelming. What an adrenaline rush. I'm just going to sit here like this until it passes." No shame or embarrassment, just truth.

Abby Paradis, "My Daughter Named the One Thing Predators Target—and the Truth of It Shook Me," *The Virago* (blog), Medium, January 29, 2026. https://medium.com.

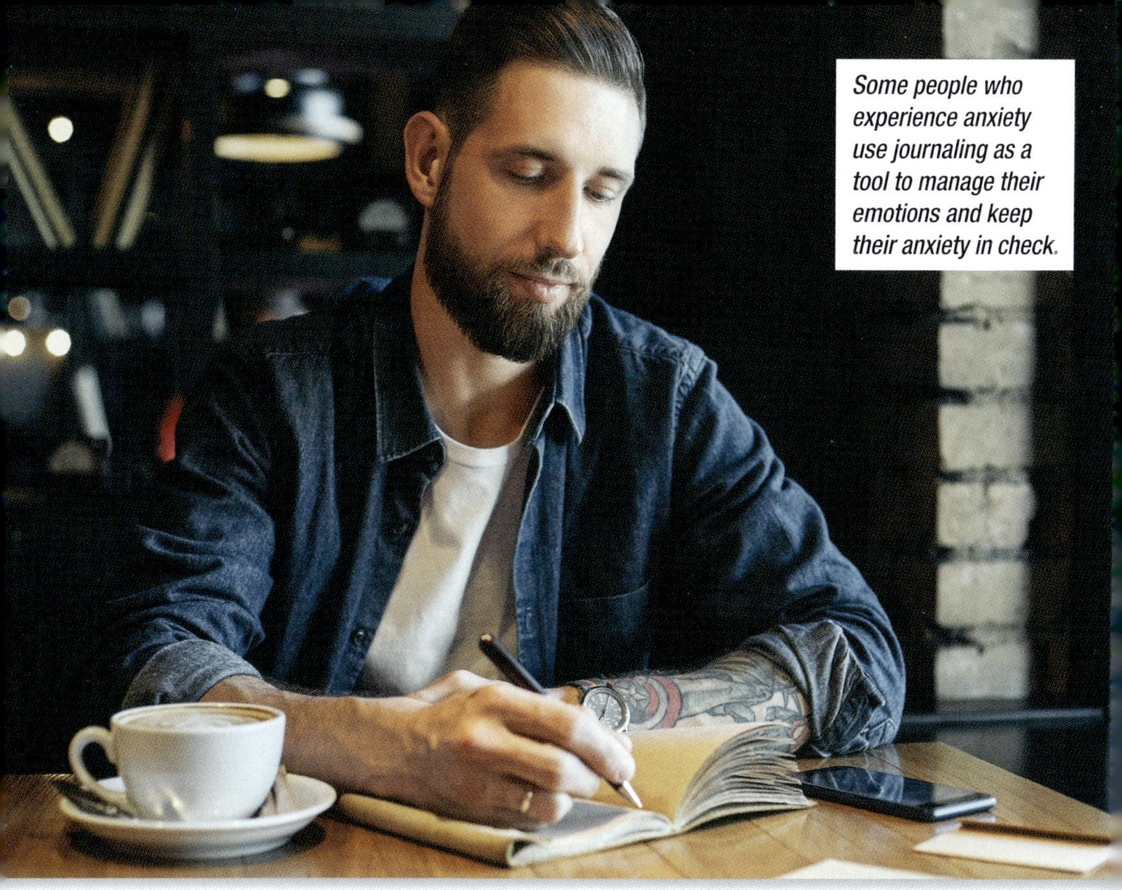

Some people who experience anxiety use journaling as a tool to manage their emotions and keep their anxiety in check.

A Lifestyle, Not a Cure

As Guschina, Beck, and Marak's stories illustrate, anxiety and panic attacks usually do not disappear completely, but they can be managed. The goal of most therapies is not to eliminate anxious feelings forever but rather to learn how to live with them in ways that keep them from taking over one's life. By focusing on management rather than a cure, people feel empowered to take control of their symptoms instead of feeling discouraged when anxiety shows up again.

One of the most powerful tools for managing anxiety is learning to recognize what sets it off. Triggers might include academic pressure, stressful social situations, family conflicts, and even phobias. Once identified, coping strategies, including deep breathing, grounding exercises, or talking to a trusted friend can help reduce the intensity of symptoms. "When panic strikes, the first line of defense is often regulating breathing," says Jennifer Barns, a writer for the website Intelligent Living. "Specific breathing techniques can provide immediate relief during a panic attack and serve as a powerful tool for managing anxiety."[31]

Barns recommends the 4-7-8 breathing method. "This simple but effective technique involves inhaling for 4 counts, holding for 7 counts, and exhaling for 8 counts. The extended exhale activates the parasympathetic nervous system, helping to calm the body's stress response. Many teens find this method particularly helpful during tests or other high-pressure situations."[32]

Healthy routines can make a big difference in how the body and mind respond to stress. Getting enough sleep helps the brain reset. Regular exercise releases chemicals that boost mood and reduce tension. Mindfulness practices, such as meditation, help people stay present instead of spiraling into worry. Eating balanced meals and limiting caffeine can also help. These proactive steps do not eliminate anxiety, but they strengthen resilience and make coping easier.

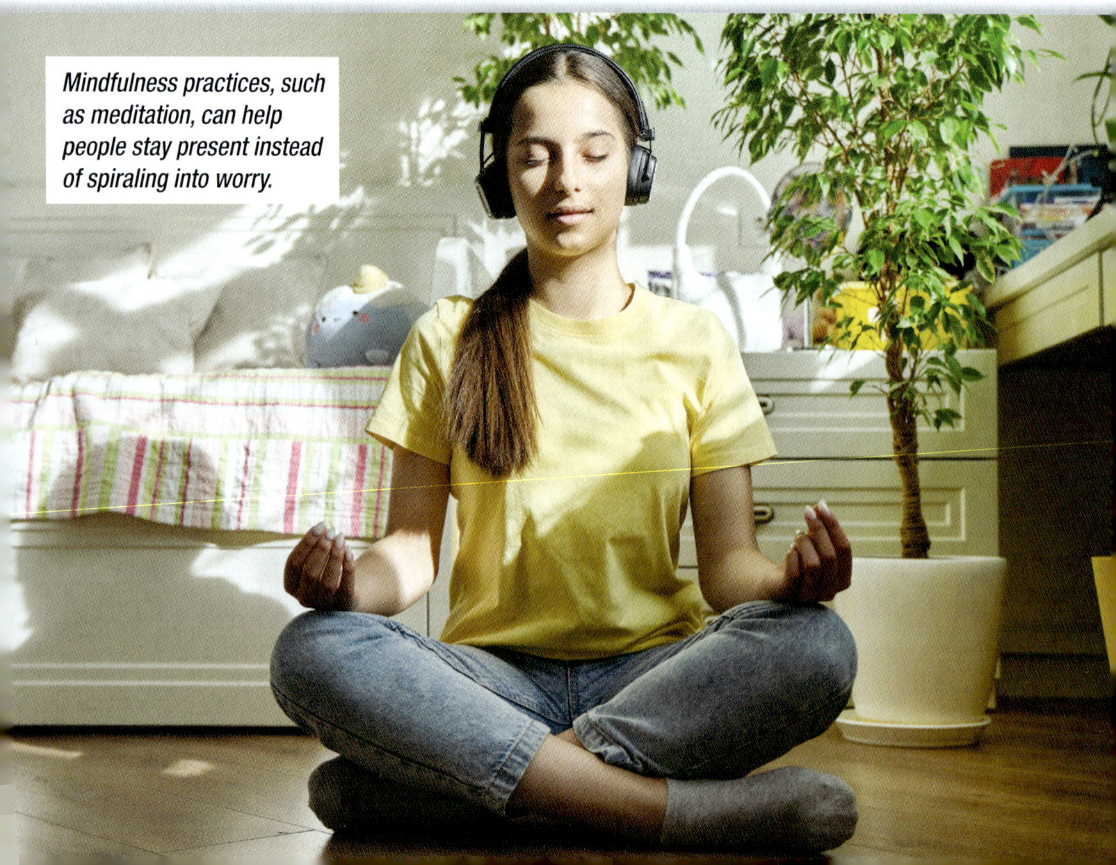

Mindfulness practices, such as meditation, can help people stay present instead of spiraling into worry.

Developing Techniques for Managing Anxiety

Annabel Lucinda, a social media influencer and the founder of Regain Your Power Apparel, a clothing company that features uplifting slogans on its products, has combined several techniques to manage her anxiety. In an October 2025 Instagram post, she explained that she was diagnosed with anxiety in 2021 after going through a traumatic event in her life. She had constant panic attacks that included depersonalization, a symptom in which the sufferer feels detached from their own body, mind, or feelings. Depersonalization is sometimes described as an "out-of-body experience," because the sufferer sometimes feels like they are watching themselves from the outside. Lucinda also experienced derealization, a symptom in which the world feels unreal, dreamlike, or distorted. This feeling is often accompanied by fear of "going crazy" or losing control. For Lucinda, these symptoms took over her life. She got to the point where she did not want to leave her apartment or even look at her phone, for fear that it would trigger a panic attack. She eventually sought professional help:

> I immediately began seeing my old therapist and she gave me a lot of great grounding exercises such as imagining myself in my "safe place," carrying around something that had a "safe smell," and breathing exercises—anything to help ground myself when needed. Although these were quick fixes, I had to address the triggers. At the time, I was living in [New York City] and constantly surrounded by triggers (people, alcohol, loud noises, etc.). I had to remove myself from my environment and find a good outlet for my anxiety which became the gym.[33]

By working out and surrounding herself with people who had a positive influence on her, Lucinda began to feel better. The anxiety-related symptoms she had been struggling with began to fade away. She continues:

> Fast forward 3 years later . . . I will very rarely have a panic attack or feel the depersonalization/derealization coming on since I'm in a much better place in my life, but it does happen from time to time. If I could give one piece of advice when it comes to anxiety, it would be to address/remove your triggers from your environment, find a good outlet (such as the gym), and be patient with yourself.[34]

Building a Support Network

Anxiety can be and usually is an isolating experience. The person feeling it is often trapped in their own mind. Many of the techniques for managing anxiety, including breathing deliberately and identifying automatic thoughts, are highly personal as well. But anxiety sufferers, especially teens, can also gain help from a net-

From Confusion to Management

Jo Ardolino is a counselor and psychotherapist. He remembers how confused he was when first diagnosed with anxiety:

> When I was a teenager, I often found myself struggling to cope with daily life. I experienced constant chest pains, tight muscles in my upper back and shoulders, stomach issues, and I was frequently sick. To manage, I turned to overeating, which caused significant weight gain and only made things worse. After many visits to different doctors, mostly for my physical symptoms, I was finally referred to a clinical psychologist. . . .
>
> When I was diagnosed with anxiety, I didn't really understand what it meant. I remember telling my parents, "So, I'm just scared? That's it? How am I supposed to explain that at school?" At that time, I had no real understanding of mental health, and getting this diagnosis felt embarrassing and disempowering. . . . But over time, with support from my family and therapy, I began to understand that anxiety was much more than just feeling "scared." It was both a mental and a physical experience. . . .
>
> Today, I have a fulfilling career, a loving family, and a life that my younger self could never have imagined.

Jo Ardolino, "Understanding Anxiety: Personal Stories," Counselling Directory, November 6, 2024. www.counselling-directory.org.uk.

work of friends who are trained to identify their particular anxiety symptoms and assist with coping strategies.

Most people are eager to help their friends, but they are not sure what to do. Turning friends and family into a support network can be as easy as teaching them to say things like "breathe deeply," "remain calm," and "stay present" when they notice that the person is growing anxious. They can also remind the sufferer that the intense feelings they are experiencing will usually pass. If the friend has been taught breathing techniques like the 4-7-8 breathing method, they can join in with the sufferer. Doing a breathing exercise together creates a bond and makes the anxiety sufferer feel less isolated.

A friend can also join the anxious person in performing a grounding technique known as the 5-4-3-2-1 method. This exercise directs the sufferer's attention to their senses by having them identify five things they can see, four things they can touch, three things they can hear, two things they can smell, and one thing they can taste. The process of searching for these things, identifying them, and numbering them interrupts the anxiety cycle and helps to ground the sufferer. Doing the exercise with a friend decreases the stigma of having anxiety and provides a pathway for the friend to be of real assistance during a stressful time.

"Sharing strategies and challenges with others who 'get it' reduces isolation and stigma while providing valuable mental health tips for teens from those with lived experience."[35]

—Jennifer Barns, writer for the website Intelligent Living

It is important for the friend to stay calm themselves and validate the sufferer's experience, instead of minimizing it with phrases like "just calm down." Discussing their anxiety issues with their friends and training them in coping strategies benefits both the anxiety sufferer and the person who gives assistance. "Sharing strategies and challenges with others who 'get it' reduces isolation and stigma while providing valuable mental health tips for teens from those with lived experience,"[35] says Barns.

The concept of a support network can be extended into the school, with the help of teachers, counselors, and administrators.

For example, a student might establish a code word that they can use to quietly alert teachers that they are feeling anxious and need to practice one of their grounding techniques. A student with anxiety can also work with school counselors to create special spaces where they can go to calm down when feeling overwhelmed. Just knowing that they have a place to go to when feeling anxious can reduce the fear of having a panic attack at school and, consequently, make them less likely to occur. In the event that a student has a panic attack, having a safe zone to go to gives them a concrete action to take during times of high anxiety.

Many Options

People now have many options for managing anxiety and panic attacks, including medications, conscious therapies like CBT and ACT, creative therapy, journaling, and lifestyle changes. Often, people combine several of these approaches. Whatever their approach, millions of people live full, meaningful lives while managing anxiety and panic attacks. They go to school, build friendships, play sports, and pursue careers. Anxiety may be part of their story, but it does not define who they are or what they can achieve. As Abby Paradis, whose fourteen-year-old daughter has anxiety, puts it, "We don't need perfection, because we're more than thrilled with manageable."[36]

Introduction: An Overwhelming Feeling

1. Judith A. Verduzco, "My First Panic Attack (and What I've Learned Since)," *Monarchs Wellness Blog*, Monarchs Therapy, September 2025. https://monarchstherapy.com.
2. Clinton Kane, "I Was Having a Panic Attack—EP 003," YouTube, June 15, 2025. www.youtube.com.
3. Mayo Clinic Staff, "Panic Attacks and Panic Disorder," Mayo Clinic, May 4, 2018. www.mayoclinic.org.

Chapter One: What Is Anxiety?

4. Glory Emmanuel, "The Day I Realized My Anxiety Wasn't Failure, It Was a Signal. Here's What Changed," *Glory's Space* (blog), Medium, December 4, 2025. https://medium.com/@GloryE/the-day-i-realized-my-anxiety-wasnt-failure-it-was-a-signal-here-s-what-changed-639519c006f9.
5. Quoted in Condor Performance, "The Best Sport Psychology Quotes," April 11, 2025. https://condorperformance.com.
6. Quoted in Peter Dewey, "Steph Curry Reveals He Suffers from Performance Anxiety Ahead of Games," Ahn Fire Digital, January 7, 2025. https://ahnfiredigital.com.
7. Nick Hobson, "Anxiety Makes Us Perform Better," *Ritual and the Brain* (blog), *Psychology Today*, September 5, 2017. www.psychologytoday.com.
8. Hobson, "Anxiety Makes Us Perform Better."
9. Easy_Quail3214, comment on lostintheworld89, "Generalized Anxiety Disorder—I'm 33 and I Have Been Suffering for Years," Anxiety subreddit, Reddit, February 2024. www.reddit.com.
10. Lenibell Marak, "Living Beyond Anxiety," Anxiety and Depression Association of America, June 24, 2025. https://adaa.org.

Chapter Two: Inside a Panic Attack

11. Ryan McCarney and Heather Eastman, "Changing the Future of Mental Health and Athletics," Personal Stories, Anxiety and Depression Association of America, October 18, 2021. https://adaa.org.
12. Annabeth Suchy, "When TV Shows like 'This Is Us' Hit on Mental Health Realities," Cleveland.com, June 4, 2017. www.cleveland.com.
13. Brynn Burger, "What an Anxiety Attack Really Feels Like," *Guest Blogs, ADDitude Magazine*, April 8, 2024. www.additudemag.com.
14. Yasmina Rebani-Lee, "Unpacking My Panic Attack," *NAMI Blog*, National Alliance on Mental Illness, May 13, 2022. www.nami.org.

15. Carinne Deeds, "Surviving Panic Disorder Is Something to Be Proud Of," *Personal Stories* (blog), National Alliance on Mental Illness, May 19, 2020. www.nami.org.
16. Deeds, "Surviving Panic Disorder Is Something to Be Proud Of."
17. Rebani-Lee, "Unpacking My Panic Attack."

Chapter Three: Causes and Triggers

18. Quoted in UNC Health, "Does Anxiety Run in Families?," *UNC Health Talk* (blog), August 11, 2020. https://healthtalk.unchealthcare.org.
19. Christine Wolkin, "My Journey with Anxiety and Panic Disorder," *Personal Stories* (blog), National Alliance on Mental Illness, October 16, 2015. www.nami.org.
20. Wolkin, "My Journey with Anxiety and Panic Disorder."
21. Suchy, "When TV Shows like 'This Is Us' Hit on Mental Health Realities."

Chapter Four: Getting Treatment

22. Kasey, "How CBT Helped Me Find Happiness," Mind.org, September 3, 2021. www.mind.org.uk.
23. Jimjamjuice69, "Finally Have an SNRI Medication Working for Me," PTSD subreddit, Reddit, March 2024. www.reddit.com.
24. South West News Service, "Gen Z Has the Hardest Time Sleeping in Silence—Here's Why," *New York Post*, February 5, 2025. https://nypost.com.

Chapter Five: Living with Anxiety and Panic Attacks

25. Tanya Guschina, "Creativity Became My Way of Balancing OCD and Anxiety," Anxiety and Depression Association of America, September 17, 2025. https://adaa.org.
26. Martha Beck, *Beyond Anxiety: Curiosity, Creativity, and Finding Your Life's Purpose*. Open Field, 2025, p. xxiv.
27. Beck, *Beyond Anxiety*, p. xx.
28. Beck, *Beyond Anxiety*, pp. xxv–xxvi.
29. Marak, "Living Beyond Anxiety."
30. Marak, "Living Beyond Anxiety."
31. Jennifer Barns, "Managing Teen Panic Attacks: Your Guide to 8 Effective Relief Strategies," Intelligent Living, May 10, 2025. www.intelligentliving.co.
32. Barns, "Managing Teen Panic Attacks."
33. Annabel Lucinda (@annabel.lucinda), "How I Manage Anxiety," Instagram, October 25, 2025. www.instagram.com/p/DQPbK_dD68y/?hl=en.
34. Lucinda, "How I Manage Anxiety."
35. Barns, "Managing Teen Panic Attacks."
36. Abby Paradis, "No Soup for You!—Medical Invalidation Hurts More than It Heals," *Parenting Portal* (blog), Medium, November 14, 2025. https://medium.com.

Books

Richard Bass, *The Teens' Workbook to Self-Regulate: Empowering Teenagers to Handle Emotions with Success Through Coping Strategies and CBT Exercises*. RBG, 2022.

Martha Beck, *Beyond Anxiety: Curiosity, Creativity, and Finding Your Life's Purpose*. Open Field, 2025.

Russell Kennedy, *Anxiety Rx: A Revolutionary New Prescription for Anxiety Relief—from the Doctor Who Created It*. St. Martin's Essentials, 2024.

Kati Morton, *Are You OK? A Guide to Caring for Your Mental Health*. HarperCollins, 2024.

Charles B. Nemeroff and W. Edward Craighead, eds., *Patient Guide to Mood and Anxiety Disorders*. American Psychiatric Association, 2024.

Internet Sources

Jennifer Barns, "Managing Teen Panic Attacks: Your Guide to 8 Effective Relief Strategies," Intelligent Living, May 10, 2025. www.intelligentliving.co.

Sheila Achar Josephs, "Helping Your Anxious Teen Cope with a Panic Attack," Anxiety and Depression Association of America, July 14, 2025. https://adaa.org.

Sabrina McCrear, "How to Navigate Anxiety for Teens and Young Adults," *Health* (blog), *U.S. News & World Report*, December 13, 2024. https://health.usnews.com.

Abby Paradis, "No Soup for You!—Medical Invalidation Hurts More than It Heals," *Parenting Portal* (blog), Medium, November 14, 2025. https://medium.com.

Websites

Anxiety and Depression Association of America (ADAA)
www.adaa.org
The ADAA is a national nonprofit organization dedicated to the prevention, treatment, and cure of anxiety, depression, and other mental health challenges. The website offers evidence-based coping strategies, personal stories, and professional resources to help teens understand and manage anxiety, depression, and other conditions.

Child Mind Institute
www.childmind.org
The Child Mind Institute provides accessible resources for teens and families on anxiety, panic attacks, and related mental health challenges.

HEARD Alliance
www.heardalliance.org
The HEARD Alliance curates trusted resources for youth, families, and educators on anxiety and related mental health issues.

Mental Health Foundation
www.mentalhealthfoundation.org
The Mental Health Foundation is focused on reducing stigma and raising awareness of mental health issues. Teens can find free, research-backed resources to manage emotions, understand mental health topics (like anxiety, depression, and bullying), and find support, including connecting with YoungMinds Crisis Messenger for immediate help.

National Alliance on Mental Illness (NAMI)
www.nami.org
NAMI is the largest grassroots mental health organization in the United States, dedicated to improving the lives of individuals and families affected by mental illness. The website hosts a large library of podcasts, webinars, and blog posts to help teens find information on a variety of mental health topics, including anxiety and panic attacks.

National Institute of Mental Health (NIMH)
www.nimh.nih.gov
Part of the National Institutes of Health, NIMH conducts and supports research to transform the understanding, treatment, and prevention of mental illnesses. The website offers reliable, research-based information on mental health topics, including depression, anxiety, stress, and eating disorders. Teens can learn about warning signs, coping strategies, and ways to seek help.

INDEX

Note: Boldface page numbers indicate illustrations.

PICTURE CREDITS

Cover: LightField Studios/Shutterstock

5: LightField Studio/Shutterstock
9: Arthur Dong/Xinhua News Agency/Newscom
11: PeopleImages/Shutterstock
14: AYO Production/Shutterstock
18: Tero Vesalainen/Shutterstock
21: Travelview/Shutterstock
24: Syda Spirit/Shutterstock
28: Photo Spirit/Shutterstock
31: PeopleImages/Shutterstock
34: Josep Suria/Shutterstock
37: AYO Production
39: wichayada suwanachun/Shutterstock
43: Hananeko_Studio/Shutterstock
49: Prostock-studio/Shutterstock
51: Shutterstock
52: Shutterstock

ABOUT THE AUTHOR

Bradley Steffens is a novelist, a poet, and an award-winning author of more than seventy-five nonfiction books for children and young adults.